LOW FODMAP RECIPES

Low Fodmap Recipes to Keep You Healthy!

(Delicious Recipe Includes Meal Plan to Soothe Your Gut)

Thomas Johnson

Published by Alex Howard

© **Thomas Johnson**

All Rights Reserved

Low Fodmap Recipes: Low Fodmap Recipes to Keep You Healthy! (Delicious Recipe Includes Meal Plan to Soothe Your Gut)

ISBN 978-1-990169-24-3

All rights reserved. No part of this guide may be reproduced in any form without permission in writing from the publisher except in the case of brief quotations embodied in critical articles or reviews.

Legal & Disclaimer

The information contained in this book is not designed to replace or take the place of any form of medicine or professional medical advice. The information in this book has been provided for educational and entertainment purposes only.

The information contained in this book has been compiled from sources deemed reliable, and it is accurate to the best of the Author's knowledge; however, the Author cannot guarantee its accuracy and validity and cannot be held liable for any errors or omissions. Changes are periodically made to this book. You must consult your doctor or get professional medical advice before using any of the suggested remedies, techniques, or information in this book.

Table of contents

Part 1 1

Chapter 1 - Fodmaps 2

What is a FODMAP diet? 2

What Are Fodmaps? 4

How Do Fodmaps Cause Symptoms? 7

What Makes The Fodmap Concept Revolutionary? 8

Which Substances Are Grouped Under The Umbrella Term 'Fodmaps'? 10

Frequently Occuring Fodmaps 15

Lactose 16

Fructose 19

Fructans 30

Galactans And Galacto-Oligosaccharides 32

Natural And Synthetic Polyols 33

CHAPTER 2: WHEN DO FODMAPS BECOME A PROBLEM? **35**

What Symptoms Do Fodmaps Cause? 35

What Happens With Fodmaps In The Small Intestine? 36

What Happens With Fodmaps In The Large Bowel? 38

Can The Fodmap Effects Be Demonstrated In Humans? 39

What End-Products Are Produced During Fermentation Of Fodmaps? 40

Are There Extra-Intestinal Fodmap Effects? 41

How Do Intestinal Gases Cause Discomfort? 42

Visceral Hypersensitivity 44

Activity Of Intestinal Muscles And Transport Velocity 46

Changes In The Intestinal Flora 46

Are The Fodmap Effects Detectable? 48

Lactulose, The Synthetic Fodmap 48

CHAPTER 3: WHO BENEFITS FROM A LOW-FODMAP DIET? 50

Which Diseases Cause Digestive Complaints? 51

CHAPTER 4: UNDERSTANDING DIETS 62

Diets For Irritable Bowel Syndrome 64

The Gradual Path To A Low-Fodmap Diet 65

What Makes The Fodmap Diet Credible? 67

Are Fodmaps Unhealthy Or Even Dangerous? 69

Is There A Risk Of Nutritional Deficiencies? 70

How Many Meals A Day Should I Eat? 70

Is The Positive Effect Of The Low-Fodmap Diet Proven? 71

Resistant Starch, Retrograded Starch: What Are They? 73

What You Should Know About Fiber 74

CHAPTER 5: THE FIRST STEP IS ALWAYS THE HARDEST 77

How Can I Reduce Fodmaps In My Diet? 79

If The Low-Fodmap Diet Does Not Help 92

What About Cheese? 93

What About Other Dairy Products? 94

What Other Foods Contain Lactose? 95

What You Should Know About Yogurt? 96

Is The Fodmap Share In Our Diet Increasing? 97

What About Meat, Fish, Chicken, Fats And Oils? 100

How To Assess The Ready-Made Products? 100

How Many Fodmaps Are In Hot Drinks? 101

How Many Fodmaps Are In Chocolate? 103

How Many Fodmaps Are Contained In Sweets And Soft Drinks? 103

How Do I Replace Onions And Garlic? 105

What Type Of Bread Is Low In Fodmaps? 106

Sweeteners 109

Spices And Herbs 110

! No Fodmap-Free Life, Please! The Handling Of Ready-To-Serve Products, Pastries And Drinks 111

Sauces And Dressings 112

Baking And Baked Goods 113

Ready-Made Gluten-Free Flour Mixtures 113

Flour Mixtures For Bread 114

Drinks 116

Is The Low-Fodmap Diet Compatible With Other Diets?? 118

Fodmaps And The Vegetarian Or Vegan Diet.. 118

PART 2 120

VEGETARIAN AND VEGAN 121

Halloumi Kebabs With Asian Dressing (Serves 2).. 122

Vegetable Tartlets (Serves 4) 125

Three Cheese Broccoli Bake (Serves 4-6).. 127

Halloumi Burgers (Serves 4) 130

Aubergine Parmigiana (Serves 4) 132

Vegetable Bake With A Cheddar And Pumpkin Crust (Serves 6) 135

Ramen With Crispy Tofu (Serves 4) 137

Vegetable Pasta Bake (Serves 4-6) 140

Griddled Courgette Salad (Serves 4) 143

Macaroni 'Cheese' (Serves 4).. 145

Whipped Feta Dip With Vegetable Crudités (Serves 4) 148

BAKING **150**

Rhubarb Cake With Lemon Sauce (Serves 8-10) 151

Strawberry Cake (Serves 6-8) 154

Gluten-Free Scones (Makes 12) 157

Lemon And Poppy Seed Pound Cake (Makes 12 Slices) 160

Palmiers (Makes 8) 163

Whoopie Pies (Makes 10) 166

Chocolate Orange Biscuits (Makes 8-10) 169

Dark Chocolate And Ginger Oaties (Makes 12) 172

Blondies (Makes 8-10) 175

Viennese Whirls (Makes 12) 178

Red Velvet Muffins (Makes 12) 181

Strawberry Turnovers (Serves 8) 184

Coffee And Walnut Cake (Serves 8-10) 186

Part 1

Chapter 1 - Fodmaps

What is a FODMAP diet?

The FODMAP diet, or rather the low-FODMAP diet, is an elimination diet based on a novel dietary approach that has been specifically developed to prevent and/or treat digestive problems. Originally, the low-FODMAP diet was developed to provide relief from the symptoms of chronic inflammatory bowel disease (IBD) such as Crohn's disease and ulcerative colitis, as well as irritable bowel syndrome. However, it can also be used in other disorders manifesting with similar digestive symptoms like in functional GI disorders (FGID). The low-FODMAP diet effectively alleviates or prevents symptoms such as bloating, flatulence, abdominal pain, soft stools, frequent bowel movements, diarrhea and constipation.

! A low-FODMAP diet means consuming foods that are low in FODMAPs, while at the same time avoiding foods high in FODMAPs. This effectively reduces gastrointestinal complaints.

The low-FODMAP diet offers relief from intestinal complaints such as bloating, diarrhea, constipation and abdominal pain.

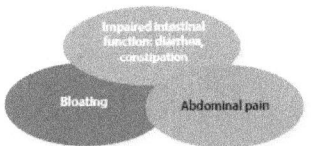

What Are Fodmaps?

FODMAPs is an English acronym for fermentable oligosaccharides, disaccharides, monosaccharides and polyols.

FODMAPs are a collection of short-chain carbohydrates and sugar alcohols that are fermentable, meaning that they are broken down (fermented) in the large bowel (colon) by enzymes derived from bacteria. All nutrients summarized under the umbrella term "FODMAPs" are found in foods naturally or as food additives.

FODMAPs are not toxic or hazardous to health, but they can contribute to the development of gastrointestinal symptoms.

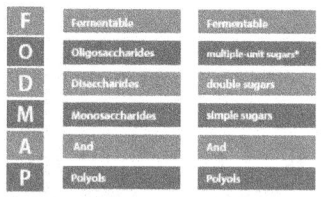

* Oligosaccharides consist of 3 to 10 monosaccharides

In 2005, a group of physicians and nutritionists from Australia hypothesized that the food, or more precisely the FODMAPs contained in the food, are responsible for the development and aggravation of GI symptoms in patients with inflammatory bowel disease. This hypothesis was based on their own observations as well as on the analysis of numerous nutritional protocols of patients with inflammatory bowel disease. These nutritional protocols revealed that the patients had consumed an excess of foods high in FODMAPs, and this observation formed the basis for the FODMAP hypothesis. FODMAPs are a broad variety of food ingredients. From a digestive viewpoint, FODMAPs have three main characteristics in common:

Absorption in the small intestine is difficult or impossible

FODMAPs are poorly or not at all absorbed in the small intestine. The reasons include the following:

- Some molecules such as polyols (sugar alcohols) are too large to pass through the intestinal wall;
- The transport capacities through the intestinal wall are limited, as is the case with fructose (fructose malabsorption);
- The enzyme activity facilitating the transport through the intestinal wall is deficient, as is the case with lactose and its corresponding enzyme lactase;
- The small intestine lacks the corresponding enzymes to hydrolyze breakdown into digestible components, as is the case with fructans (fructo-oligosaccharides) and galactans (galacto-oligosaccharides).

High water-binding capacity
In technical terms, FODMAPs are said to have a very high water-binding capacity. FODMAPs are small molecules which can bind a large amount of water. This causes fluid to accumulate in the intestine and in turn leads to an increased transport speed in the intestine with frequent bowel movements and softer stools, including diarrhea.

Rapid fermentation by gut bacteria
All FODMAPs are rapidly fermented by bacteria resident in the gut. The exact rate of bacterial fermentation depends on the length of the carbohydrate chains. FODMAPs are all short-chained and hence rapidly fermented. As a result, they trigger symptoms rather quickly.

Are all carbohydrates FODMAPs?
Carbohydrates come in a variety of forms in foods, namely as simple carbohydrates, which include monosaccharides (simple sugars) such as glucose and fructose and disaccharides (double sugars) such as sucrose and lactose, as well as complex carbohydrates (polysaccharides). The latter are further subdivided into short-chain and long-chain polysaccharides. Long-chain polysaccharides, in turn, include digestible starch and non-digestible polysaccharides such as cellulose, the structural component of the primary cell wall of

green plants. Carbohydrates are an important part of our diet. Most FODMAPs are carbohydrates, but not all carbohydrates are FODMAPs. FODMAP-carbohydrates are a well-defined group of short-chain carbohydrates. Most foods high in FODMAPs contain short-chain carbohydrates, which are poorly absorbed in the small intestine.

How Do Fodmaps Cause Symptoms?

FODMAPs are short-chain carbohydrates and sugar alcohols, which are moderately to scarcely digestible and therefore reach the colon via the small intestine in a nearly undigested form. In the colon, FODMAPs are subsequently fermented by the intestinal bacteria, also called intestinal flora. FODMAPs are decomposed during fermentation. This produces energy and various degradation products, including many gases such as hydrogen. These gases that accumulate in the intestine cause symptoms, especially bloating and flatulence. Both symptoms are reported very frequently by patients with irritable bowel syndrome, but also by those with other GI disorders. Since FODMAPs are inevitably a part of any balanced diet, the FODMAP theory assumes that patients who develop digestive complaints display specific characteristics: On the one hand, the ingestion of FODMAPs with food intake is increased; on the other hand, however, the small intestine of these patients can absorb less FODMAPs. These two causes can be present separately or in combination, with the inevitable consequence of a higher amount of FODMAPs reaching the colon.

What Makes The Fodmap Concept Revolutionary?

The fact that individual FODMAPs such as lactose, fructose or sweeteners cause symptoms is not new knowledge. For decades, we have been aware of the resulting symptoms of diarrhea and bloating. In the past, individual diets with a reduced content of lactose, fructose or gluten have been described as possibly helpful for patients with irritable bowel syndrome. All these diets assume that one or more food ingredients are responsible for the symptoms, and that the symptoms improve when fewer of these food ingredients are ingested. However, all these diets have proven inefficient or - at best minimally efficient in reducing the symptoms in patients suffering from irritable bowel syndrome.
The revolutionary aspect of the FODMAP concept is that a single diet now captures all these small

molecules rather than individual ones. The objective of this diet is not to completely eliminate all FODMAPs, but rather the concept proposes to control and reduce the amount of FODMAPs as much as possible. The goal is to reduce the total amount of FODMAPs in the food we consume to such an extent that the remaining FODMAPs no longer cause any symptoms.

! A low-FODMAP diet does not eliminate solely individual substances that may cause GI complaints; rather, it reduces all substances causing symptoms. The goal is to significantly reduce the total amount of FODMAPs.

The FODMAP theory does not mean to suggest that FODMAPs are a root cause of diseases. Irritable bowel syndrome and chronic inflammatory bowel diseases have other causes - it is not due to the FODMAP content in our food. Rather, the FODMAP theory assumes that FODMAPs are involved in the development of symptoms, particularly in the case of an existing disease and in the case of existing digestive complaints, i.e. the annoying bloating, soft stools, diarrhea and intestinal cramps.
Therefore, the goal of a low-FODMAP diet is not to treat the root cause of irritable bowel syndrome, but rather to offer a way of eventually reducing and/or avoiding symptoms. This is highly relevant and

progressive as previous IBS diets were always tailored around the presumed pathological digestion or intolerances, such as lactose or fructose intolerance.

FODMAPs are present in the food we consume and they are delivered to the colon -- that is completely normal. It is also normal that these FODMAPs are fermented in the colon by bacteria. Gastrointestinal symptoms, however, are effectively reduced if the absolute quantity of FODMAPs entering the colon is reduced by means of a consistent dietary change.

Which Substances Are Grouped Under The Umbrella Term 'Fodmaps'?

The term 'FODMAPs' encompasses fermentable oligosaccharides, disaccharides and monosaccharides as well as polyols. FODMAPs are contained in almost all foodstuffs, and you will learn more about individual FODMAPs and the FODMAP content of different foods. The first step is to become familiar with FODMAPs and to understand which FODMAPs are contained in various foodstuffs. Later, you will learn how this concept can be translated into a relevant diet. The terms oligosaccharides, disaccharides, monosaccharides and polyols do not mean much to most people. We do not automatically associate any

food ingredients with these terms. Therefore, it is important to recognize to what specific food ingredients these terms refer.
The terms oligosaccharides, disaccharides and monosaccharides refer to multiple-unit sugars, double sugars and simple sugars, respectively. The table shows which substances belong to the individual groups, and which foods contain them.

FODMAPs: An Overview

Oligosaccharides
Appear in the diet as....
Fructans, Galactans, Fructo-oligosaccharides (FOS), Galacto-oligosaccharides (GOS) Are abundantly contained in...
Barley, rye, wheat, peas, garlic, leeks, lentils, onions

Disaccharides
Appear in the diet as....
Lactose
Are abundantly contained in... Yogurt, milk, cream

Monosaccharides

Appear in the diet as....
Fructose
Are abundantly contained in...
Apples, pears, honey, cherries, corn sirup, asparagus

Polyols
Appear in the diet as.... Sorbitol (Sorbit), Mannitol (Mannit), Maltitol (Maltit), Xylitol (Xylit) Are abundantly contained in... Apples, pears, cherries, nectarines, plums, diet products, chewing gum, sweeteners

Oligosaccharides
Oligosaccharides are various sugars composed of at least three sugar molecules. All oligosaccharides are therefore carbohydrates.
Depending on how many monosaccharides the oligosaccharides are composed of, they are referred to as

- Trisaccharides (three molecules of monosaccharides),
- Tetrasaccharides (four molecules of monosaccharides), or
- Pentasaccharides (five molecules of monosaccharides).

This designation based on the exact number could be continued. It is, however, unusual to use this exact counting method.
For simplification purposes, the term oligosaccharides is often used for sugars consisting of 3 to 10 monosaccharides. Longer carbohydrate chains, i.e. those containing more than 10 aligned

monosaccharides, are called polysaccharides (multiple-unit sugars), and they play no role in the FODMAP diet. Fructans, galactans and galacto-oligosaccharides are oligosaccharides (multiple-unit sugars) that are relevant for the FODMAP concept. Fructans, which also include fructooligosaccharides (FOS), are short-chain carbohydrates consisting of very short chains of several fructose molecules and a glucose molecule at the end of the chain. Galactans are short branched-chain carbohydrates composed of individual galactose molecules. Galacto-oligosaccharides (GOS), on the other hand, are short-chain carbohydrates with chains of several galactose molecules and a glucose molecule at the end of the chain. All these oligosaccharides occur naturally and are standard food components.

Disaccharides

Disaccharides (double sugars)
High in FODMAPs: Lactose
Low in FODMAPs: Cellobiose, Gentobiose, Isomaltose, Kojibiose, Maltose, Nigerose, Primverose, Rutinose, Sucrose, Trehalose

'Disaccharide' is the technical term for a double sugar. There are numerous dissacharides which we take in with food and which are well-digested by our intestines or insignificant for symptom generation and therefore do not play any role in the FODMAP diet. The table lists various disaccharides that are ingested with food, of which lactose is relevant for the FODMAP diet.

Monosaccharides

Monosaccharides are simple sugars. Simple sugars act as energy carriers in foods and are formed in a myriad of variations in our metabolism. The simple sugar fructose is the only sugar from the group of monosaccharides that is relevant for the FODMAP diet. Other simple sugars that we take in with foodstuffs such as glucose, galactose, mannose, xylose and arabinose play no role in the FODMAP diet.

Polyols

From a chemical perspective, polyols are polyhydric alcohols. These alcohols are present in natural foodstuffs in various forms. Polyols occur naturally in a wide variety of fruits and vegetables, and provide the taste and texture of sugar with about half the calories.

Natural foods containing polyols

Mannitol: Seaweed, Mushrooms
Sorbitol: Apple, Apricot, Pear, Peach, Plum, Large amounts in dried fruits

Due to their sweet taste, these polyols are very often used by the food industry as sugar substitutes. Sorbitol, mannitol and xylitol, as well as the names of many other polyols or their corresponding European EXXX numbers for the labeling of food additives, can be found in the list of ingredients of many foodstuffs. For a detailed listing of polyols and food additive names, please refer to the table in this book. You will be surprised by the widespread presence of polyols in our foods, as well as in other products such as toothpaste or mouthwash. Due to the desire for a calorie-reduced nutrition, the proportion of polyols in our diet is increasing exponentially.

Frequently Occuring Fodmaps

The list of FODMAPs contains some well-known food ingredients occurring regularly and in large quantities in our food, such as lactose (milk sugar), fructose (fruit sugar), variations of fructose such as fructans and galacto-oligosaccharides, and some polyols.

Lactose content in dairy products:

Very high in lactose, more than 10 g /100 g: Creamer, Condensed milk, Milk powder, Whey cheese, Whey powder

High in lactose, 4-10 g /100 g: Buttermilk, Ice cream, Coffee creamer, Skimmed milk, Milk chocolate, Whey, Whole milk

Moderate lactose content, 1-4 g /100 g: Cream cheese, Cottage cheese, Yogurt, Kefir, Low-fat curd, Nut-nougat cream, Curd, Sour cream, Whipped cream
Hardly any lactose, Less than 1 g /100 g: Brie cheese, Butter, Camembert cheese, Feta cheese, Hard cheese

Since these are food ingredients that are present in our usual diet, and quite notably in a healthy diet, it is a good idea to examine these food components more closely. This will help you recognize what to look for and how to shape your future diet.

Lactose

Also referred to as "milk sugar," lactose is a disaccharide, composed of the monosaccharide components glucose and galactose. In our intestine, the enzyme lactase breaks down lactose into two monosaccharides. Only after this decomposition can the two monosaccharide components be absorbed into the bloodstream through the intestinal wall and used as energy carriers. Humans are born naturally able to produce ample amounts of lactase in order to digest mother's milk that is very rich in lactose while nursing. Lactase activity in the intestine decreases with age since we do not feed on mother's milk for a lifetime, and the consumption of milk and dairy products decreases with advancing age.

In regions like Europe where dairy products are consumed for a lifetime, there is higher intestinal lactase activity in adults than in regions where dairy products are not consumed, such as in Africa or Southeast Asia. In western societies, approximately two-thirds of adults still have measurable intestinal lactase activity, while the remaining one-third have no measurable lactase activity. The figures below show the extent of this distinctive geographic distribution of lactase activity in adults. While 98% of adults in the Scandinavian countries have a detectable intestinal lactase activity, only less than 10% of adults in Africa or Asia have a measurable lactase activity. For most people, the intestinal lactase activity is irrelevant, since the diet in the adult age is no longer based exclusively on dairy products. Rather, it includes merely low amounts of dairy products. Precisely because our diet contains little lactose, a diminished or an altogether absent lactase activity in the intestine is insignificant for most people in the adult age.
Lactose, which is not broken down in the small intestine because there is insufficient enzyme or enzyme activity, cannot be absorbed into the bloodstream from the intestine. Unchanged, the lactose enters the colon where it is then fermented by colonic bacteria, giving rise to bacterial degradation products, including many gases which in turn can cause

discomfort.

For this reason, the lack of lactase activity is revealed in some adults when they get GI complaints, especially when their diet contains many dairy products. A diet that is rich in dairy products is generally not unhealthy if one tolerates it well. The symptoms caused by lactose can range from occasional mild symptoms to frequent and severe symptoms. In the case of frequent symptoms that seem to be induced by lactose, a physician should be consulted to check for lactose intolerance. If confirmed, special dietary recommendations should be considered.

! When eating foods high in lactose induces symptoms on a regular basis, a physician should be consulted to check for lactose intolerance.

What foods contain lactose?
The "milk sugar" lactose is contained in all dairy products such as milk, cheese, yogurt and curd. Normal cow's milk, for example, contains between 4 and 8 % lactose. The exact lactose content varies depending on the origin of the milk; cow's milk, for example, has a different lactose content than sheep milk, goat milk or horse milk. Lactose is found in all dairy products, but in varying amounts depending on how the dairy product has been further processed. The lactose table in this book shows the lactose content of different dairy

products.

A lesser-known but interesting fact is that lactose is often added as a stabilizer or flavoring agent in industrially processed foods. Therefore, you should always read the list of ingredients of processed foods carefully to see where lactose has been added. Furthermore, lactose is found in numerous medications as a diluent or filler, since lactose is very cost effective and inherently compactable, that is, able to form a solid compact (i.e. tablet) under compression. However, the lactose content of medicinal products should not be taken into account due to the very small amounts.

Lactose is found in varying amounts in all dairy products. It is also used as a stabilizer and flavoring agent in other foods.

Fructose

Fructose is a simple sugar with a very high sweetness level. It is found naturally in herbal products. Foods naturally rich in fructose include honey, raisins and other dried fruits. Fructose is extracted from sugar cane, sugar beet or corn. In addition to glucose, all three plants contain high amounts of fructose. Owing to its high sweetness level, simple extraction and, in some cases also due to its brown color, fructose is often added to food and beverages. Information on the fructose content of each food is indicated in the list of ingredients.

There are several reasons why fructose is poorly or not at all absorbed in the small intestine. It may be that too much fructose is contained in the food, the food is transported too rapidly through the small intestine, or that the number of the intestinal fructose transporters (GLUT-5) is too low or their activity too weak.

! When eating foods high in fructose induces symptoms on a regular basis, a physician should be consulted to check for fructose malabsorption.

Breath hydrogen testing can be used to detect malabsorption of fructose, i.e. a restricted fructose uptake. Alternative terms for fructose malabsorption are dietary fructose intolerance or intestinal fructose intolerance

A completely different disease is hereditary fructose intolerance, a very rare hereditary metabolic disease. This disease is detected by genetic testing. Due to all these various terms, one must carefully consider which disorder is exactly meant.

Ways of fructose absorption
Since fructose is a simple sugar, it does not have to be broken down in the intestine before it can be absorbed

into the bloodstream. It is first taken as a whole from the intestine by the intestinal absorptive cells (enterocytes) and then released from them into the bloodstream. This uptake and release of fructose by the enterocytes is regulated by a special transport protein located in the cell walls. The transport protein for fructose is named GLUT-5. Usually, fructose is completely absorbed across the intestine into the bloodstream. Fructose digestion becomes a problem only when there is too much fructose in the intestine. In such a case, the absorptive capacity of the body may become exhausted and the transport function of GLUT-5 overloaded. As a consequence, fructose is incompletely absorbed into the bloodstream from the small intestine and it enters the colon.

! For various reasons, modern-day diets can contain very high amounts of fructose. In a normal, balanced diet, fructose content often exceeds the absorptive capacity of our bodies.

The intestine can absorb approximately 35-50 g of fructose per day using the fructose transporter. The average daily amount of consumed fructose (50-60 g) already slightly exceeds the normal uptake capacity of a human being. Since these figures indicate the average intake, it is very clear that in many people the fructose intake with their diet significantly exceeds the uptake capacity of the intestine. However, fructose uptake from the intestine into the body is subject to a few additional properties. For one, the fructose transporter Glut-5 can be blocked by polyols like sorbitol. Therefore, a diet rich in sorbitol (e.g. consuming sorbitol-rich plums) results in a diminished fructose uptake in the intestine. Furthermore, diseases such as hypertension, diabetes and obesity can diminish fructose uptake, because these diseases are associated by an impaired activity of the fructose transporter. It is exactly the opposite in the presence of glucose. The presence of glucose in the intestine facilitates the uptake of fructose. That is why fruit containing a balanced ratio of fructose and glucose is better digestible than fruit that is naturally rich in fructose.

What happens to fructose in the colon? Fructose, which is not absorbed in the small intestine, enters the colon where it is fermented by the intestinal bacteria or fungi (yeasts). This results in bacterial degradation products and gases such as carbon dioxide, which can cause discomfort. In contrast to the long-chain fructans and galactans, the fermentation of fructose is faster, meaning that the intake of fructose leads to symptoms more rapidly.

What makes fructose so attractive to food processing industry?

There are several reasons why fructose is often used in industrially processed foods. One reason is certainly the high sweetness value of fructose. Compared to glucose, fructose is two and a half times sweeter. This difference is even greater when compared to lactose fructose is eleven times sweeter than lactose. In view of this, it is easy to understand why fructose is the preferred agent in industrial food processing.

However, there are other reasons for the use of fructose. Sometimes, fructose is used in industrial food processing since it can form chemical compounds with the proteins contained in the foods. The advantage of these compounds is the formation of a light brownish discoloration; hence, in this context, fructose can be referred to as a sweetener and food coloring agent. Fructose is used as a food coloring agent when a light brown color of the resulting product is desired such as in bread and other pastries. Furthermore, fructose is used in beverage production. Yeasts used in the production of alcoholic beverages can ferment fructose as well as glucose. Such fructose-containing drinks have a slightly higher residual sweetness and are also suitable for diabetics in limited amounts. The desired end-products are alcohol and carbon dioxide, which initially remains dissolved in the beverage and is released only upon opening the bottle.

Foods high in fructose content
Dried fruits: Apple, Pear, Date, Mango, Raisins/sultanas
Fresh fruits: Apple, Pear, Fig, Persimmon (kaki), Cherry, Mango
Cereals: Crunchy honey flakes, Honeygranola/muesli
Other foods: Products for diabetics, Fruit concentrates, Fruit juice, Instant beverages, Honey, Invert sugar sirup

What is the significance of the ratio of glucose to fructose?
In connection with the fructose content of fruits, the sucrose content of these foods is also important, since the disaccharide sucrose is broken down into the simple sugars glucose and fructose. For this reason, sucrose too has to be regarded as a source of fructose.

! The glucose-to-fructose ratio in foods plays a very significant role in the assessment of their tolerability. A ratio greater than 1 (> 1) implies more glucose than fructose and hence a better tolerability. Some examples can be found in the table in this book.

! A ratio less than 1 (< 1) implies more fructose than glucose and hence a poorer tolerability.
! On the whole, however, the glucose-to-fructose ratio plays a less significant role than the absolute fructose content.

Fruits contain fructose and sucrose in different amounts. Apples and pears, for example, are extremely rich in fructose, while apricots and peaches are low in fructose. Fructose is also contained in products which we do not immediately associate with the term fructose, such as honey or molasses, i.e. sugar beet sirup. Both are products that can be consumed on their own as spreads, or as additions to other foods (sweeteners). Corn syrup, for instance, is very complex when it comes to considering its fructose content. It is frequently found in the list of ingredients of foods and is used as a sweetener. In its inherent form, corn syrup consists mainly of glucose. In food processing industry, however, it can be treated enzymatically, so that the glucose contained in it is converted into fructose. Such enzymatically-treated corn syrup is referred to as glucose-fructose syrup (the German term) or high-fructose corn syrup (HFCS) (the English term). This enzymatic conversion is advantageous since fructose has a higher sweetening level at the same sugar quantity. The fructose content in corn syrup can be increased to a maximum of 90%.

The European Union Sugar Directive from 2001 states that any sugar sirup with at least a 5% fructose content must be declared as a glucose-fructose syrup or fructose-glucose syrup.

Glucose-fructose ratio of selected fruits and honey

unfavorably: Apple, 0.4; Apple, dried, 0.4; Mango, 0.3; Pear, 0.2; Watermelon, 0.5 **favorably:** Pineapple, 0.9; Blueberry, 0.7; Strawberry, 1.0; Raspberry, 0.8; Currant, 0.8; Kiwi, 1.0; Orange, 0.9; Peach, 0.8; Gooseberry, 0.9; Honey, 0.9

Is an increased fructose content in the diet damaging to health?
In small quantities, fructose is not unhealthy as it is a naturally-occurring sugar. Neither a carcinogenic nor a mutagenic effect of fructose has been reported thus far. However, the consumption of fructose is nevertheless associated with some risks. Glucose is

absorbed by the body and then consumed or stored in the metabolism under the control of the body's hormone insulin.
Fructose is also absorbed from the intestine into the bloodstream and reaches the liver where it is introduced into the body's metabolism, independently of the body's insulin, i.e. in a somewhat uncontrolled manner. Therefore, fructose is said to have negative effects on our health, especially when the fructose intake is very high. Excessive fructose consumption is presumably a cause of obesity (an excessive weight gain), fatty liver disease, the dangerous insulin resistance (a precursor to diabetes), as well as of the metabolic syndrome and disorders of lipid metabolism. Furthermore, it is assumed that fructose does not induce a feeling of satiety to the same extent as glucose does, a further mechanism that leads to an increased hunger sensation and ultimately to weight gain. There are significant gaps in our current understanding of fructose and much remains speculative at the moment. There are, however, very clear indications from medical research that our bodies cannot handle fructose as well as glucose. This should not be a problem for people who eat normally that is to say for those who do not consume excessive amounts and have no malabsorption issues. The unfavorable metabolic properties of fructose become

problematic only when the fructose content in the diet increases too much, as is currently the case.

! The consumption of refined fructose has risen strongly with the consumption of industrially processed foods.

Why is the fructose content in our diet increasing?
The answers to the previous questions have already indicated that fructose offers advantages over glucose in industrial food processing and is therefore increasingly contained in our foods in terms of quantity and spectrum of foods.
However, this is not the only reason why the fructose content in our diet is steadily increasing. Another reason is that our diet should be increasingly healthy and we are supposed to eat healthier foods. But much of what appears healthy at first sight is, when studied closely, not as healthy as we thought.
For instance, a fruit bar has a much higher fructose content than the consumption of the comparable quantity of fresh fruit. Another very clear example is that a glass of apple juice, which contains the best of four apples, naturally also contains the fructose quantity of four apples.

! The fructose content in our diet has increased exponentially. In some people, the gastrointestinal tract cannot cope with this excess supply of fructose, resulting in symptoms.

In many people, the gastrointestinal tract handles it well, but in some people, the gastrointestinal tract cannot cope with this excess supply of fructose, and symptoms develop, particularly when the intestine is additionally overloaded with an excess of other FODMAPs.

To what extent is fructose consumption increasing? For the European population, there are currently no good figures on the average daily fructose consumption. Old estimates predict that an adult in central Europe will take in an average of 50-60 g of fructose per day. This corresponds to approximately 20 kg of fructose per year. There are far better estimates on the sugar consumption of refined (i..e. industrially processed) sugar in the United States of America. The total sugar consumption has risen from 40 kg of sugar per capita per year in the seventies of the last century to a current 50 kg of refined sugar. It is interesting to note that the consumption of refined fructose was less than 1 kg per capita per year in the seventies, while now it is as high as 20 kg per capita per year. This amount of refined fructose is consumed via the industrially processed foods in addition to our consumption of natural fructose. From these numbers it becomes clear that the strong rise in fructose in our diet is caused primarily by the industrially processed foodstuffs.

Fructans

Fructans (fructo-oligosaccharides/FOS and fructo-polysaccharides) are multi-unit sugars consisting of a glucose ring and at least two fructose rings. Fructans with less than ten fructose rings are called fructo-oligosaccharides, and fructans with more than ten fructose rings are called inulins. In addition to starch and sucrose, fructans are the most important herbal carbohydrate stores. In addition to plants, some bacteria and yeasts can also produce and store fructans.

Fructans occur naturally in a variety of foods such as, characteristically, onions which are high in fructans. Substantial quantities of fructans are also found in cereals, beetroot, tubers and sprouts. A very high content of fructans is also found in topinambur tubers and chicory roots. The fructan content varies depending on the cultivation conditions such as season, temperature and precipitation.

Foods high in fructans: Artichoke, Chicory root, Cereals (barley, rye, wheat), Garlic, Topinambur (tubers), Leek, Beetroot, Asparagus, Onion

The names of fructans are hardly known; on occasion, the terms 'levans' and 'inulins' are found on food packaging. The table in this book shows a list of foods high in fructans. Chicory is very interesting as it is used not only as a salad, but also for the production of coffee, or, more precisely, substitute coffee. This substitute coffee is known as 'country coffee', 'chicory root coffee' or 'carob coffee', as well as 'chicory water' in Austria.

What happens to fructans in the intestine?
The human small intestine does not produce enzymes capable of hydrolyzing fructans, and as such they cannot be absorbed across the small intestine. Therefore, they are delivered to the large bowel. Due to their indigestibility, fructans are used to a small extent as additives for dietary and diabetic products. Therefore, fructans are often listed in the lists of ingredients of these products. Fructans are used as additives as they are considered calorie-free dietary fiber.

These added fructans are to be considered for a FODMAP diet. On average, we consume about 10 g of fructans daily. The human body can handle this amount well. They are broken down by the colonic bacteria, and various degradation products, especially gases, develop, just as in the case of lactose and fructose entering the colon. Since fructans may be both short-chained or long-chained, some fructans are associated with a more rapid development of symptoms than others.

Galactans And Galacto-Oligosaccharides

Galactans and galacto-oligosaccharides are carbohydrates consisting of several sugar rings. Galacto-oligosaccharides are simple chains of up to eight sugar rings, while galactans are branched chains. At least one of these sugar rings is the simple sugar galactose, from which galactans got their name.

Foods high in galacto-oligosaccharides and galactans: **Beans, Chickpeas, Lentils, Soy beverages**

Galacto-oligosaccharides are natural ingredients of numerous foods. Typical galactooligosaccharides are raffinose, a triple-unit sugar consisting of fructose, glucose and galactose, and stachyose, a four-unit sugar consisting of fructose, glucose and two galactose rings. Large amounts of these galacto-oligosaccharides are found in legumes such as beans, lentils and soybean. Galactans occur naturally mainly in the plant cell walls. Because of their gel-forming properties, galactans are frequently used in food processing as thickening or gelling agents. Frequently used galactans are carrageenans from algae (E 407), agar agar (E 406) and tragacanth, a natural polysaccharide produced from the tree Astralagus gummifer (E 413). Like other FODMAPs, galacto-oligosaccharides and galactans cannot be absorbed or digested in our intestine since the available enzymes cannot hydrolyze the bonds between the sugar rings in these chains.

Natural And Synthetic Polyols

Sugar alcohols, or polyols, are a group of ingredients that are used as sugar substitutes in our diet. The most well-known polyols are mannitol and sorbitol. The name designation is in some cases somewhat confusing i.e. sorbitol is also known as hexanhexol or glucitol. For all other polyolstheir names usually end with –ol like mannitol or xylitol. These sugar substitutes are mostly produced synthetically and in the European Union they are additionally labeled with an E number for food additives (E XXX). You will find a list of polyols below.

In North America, many foods such as sweets and, in particular, chewing gum, are often labeled with health warnings, which indicate that polyols contained may cause diarrhea, as gum addicts will readily confirm.

Polyols and their E numbers for food additive labeling
Erythritol, E 968
Isomaltol, E 953

Lactitol, E 966
Maltitol, E 965
Mannitol, E 421
Sorbitol, E 420
Xylitol, E 967

Polyols also occur naturally. A relatively large amount of sorbitol is for example found in apples, pears, plums and peaches. Polyols are hardly metabolized in the small intestine or absorbed across the small intestine and are thus delivered to the colon in an undigested form. Like other FODMAPs, they too are fermented by colonic bacteria.

Chapter 2: When Do Fodmaps Become A Problem?

What Symptoms Do Fodmaps Cause?

FODMAPs, or rather an excess of FODMAPs, mainly cause digestive problems. Various studies revealed that a diet high in FODMAPs can worsen symptoms, while a diet low in FODMAPs alleviates symptoms. Digestive symptoms aggravated by FODMAPs include bloating, flatulence, abdominal pain, diarrhea, constipation, heartburn, and nausea. Interestingly, several studies showed that even fatigue, decreased drive, lethargy, and a poor mood improved when switching to a low-FODMAP diet. This is most likely due to the fact that digestive problems affect the entire body. Noteworthy, the improvements achieved by a low-FODMAP diet are at least as good as the improvements brought about by medications or probiotic treatments.

! An excess in FODMAPs leads to digestive symptoms, most notably to bloating, flatulence, abdominal pain, diarrhea, constipation and heartburn, but also to fatigue and lethargy.

Does everyone get symptoms from FODMAPs?
No. Although FODMAPs are poorly digested by all

people -- the healthy and patients with digestive problems alike -- not all people develop symptoms. Symptoms tend to occur only in some people, more precisely in those with a particularly sensitive and susceptible gut.

The line here is rather fuzzy, which means that healthy people too can occasionally experience flatulence, increased intestinal gas, or loose stools. If this occurs only occasionally, it is not really a problem... There's more than a grain of truth in the wellknown sentence "Every little bean will make its own little sound" (referring to flatulence related to consumption of legumes).

Why do FODMAPs cause symptoms in some people?
The reasons why some people experience symptoms after consuming FODMAPs include:

- intestinal hypersensitivity, i.e. a sensitive gut;
- a change in the activity of the intestinal muscles and hence a modified transport speed, and
- a change in the composition of the bacteria resident in the intestine resulting in a modification of intestinal gas formation caused by FODMAPs.

What Happens With Fodmaps In The Small Intestine?

In the small intestine, FODMAPs are neither digested nor absorbed, but they are rather transported directly into the colon in an unchanged form. During this transport, FODMAPs bind water in the small intestine. This water binding is called osmotic activity. The increased water bound in the intestine contributes to diarrhea, while the increased formation of gas in the small intestine causes abdominal pain since the small intestine is particularly sensitive.

In addition, it is believed that small intestinal bacterial overgrowth and altered intestinal microbiota are features in patients with irritable bowel syndrome (IBS). This colonization of the small intestine with harmful bacteria leads to earlier and more intense triggering of the symptoms caused by FODMAPs after food intake, since additional intestinal gases can arise earlier in the digestion process, namely already in the small intestine. In fact, there is convincing evidence that an altered bacterial colonization of the small intestine occurs more frequently in IBS patients than in the unaffected population. However, a direct relationship between the altered intestinal microbiota in these patients and the development of symptoms by increased FODMAP intake with food has not yet been conclusively established.

What Happens With Fodmaps In The Large Bowel?

In the large intestine (colon), FODMAPs are fermented by the resident bacteria. This process generates intestinal gases and other degradation products. The intestinal gases lead to bloating, flatulence and abdominal pain. There are short-chain and long-chain FODMAPs. Short-chain FODMAPs are fermented much more quickly by the intestinal bacteria than the long-chain ones, meaning that fermentation of lactose, for instance, leads to the generation of intestinal gases much faster than fermentation of long-chain FODMAPs.

Mechanisms of symptom generation by FODMAPs

Small intestine:
Increased gas formation ---> pain, bloating, flatulence
Increased water binding ---> loose stools, rapid transport, diarrhea

Large intestine (colon):
Increased gas formation ---> pain, bloating, flatulence
Increased water binding ---> loose stools, rapid transport, diarrhea
Increased stool mass---> rapid transport, nausea

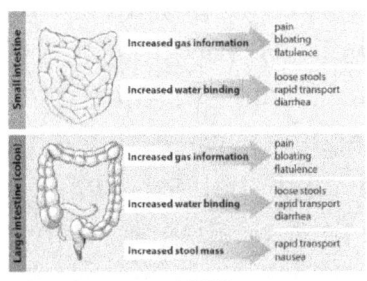

Mechanisms of symptom generation by FODMAPs

In addition, fermentation of FODMAPs in the colon produces degradation products which bind water in the intestine and actively cause the intestinal mucosa to release water into the intestine. Both mechanism lead to loose stools, including diarrhea. Fermentation in the colon, and the resulting degradation products, cause additional issues such as partial alteration of the intestinal bacterial flora, changes in the colorectal mucosa cells and inflammatory processes in the colonic wall, resulting in increased permeability of the colon's wall. This increased permeability, in turn, promotes inflammatory processes of the colorectal wall.

Can The Fodmap Effects Be Demonstrated In Humans?

A diet high in FODMAPs leads to an increase in intestinal gasses and hence an increase in flatulence and digestive problems. A scientific study has shown this to hold true for the patients with irritable bowel syndrome as well as for unaffected persons. It is interesting to note that the amount of intestinal gas produced by a high-FODMAP diet is the same in both healthy people and patients with irritable bowel syndrome, but the patients report more severe symptoms and a more pronounced flatulence. This phenomenon is explained by the hypersensitive gut in patients with IBS. Also interesting is the fact that the intestinal flora in people who consume a diet high in FODMAPs is more strongly altered in IBS patients than in unaffected people. The significance of these changes in the intestinal microbiota is still unclear.

What End-Products Are Produced During Fermentation Of Fodmaps?

Fermentation of FODMAPs produces gases, short-chain fatty acids and lactic acid. The resulting gases are mainly hydrogen (H_2) and carbon dioxide (CO_2). Other gases like ammonia (NH_3), oxygen (O_2), methane (CH_4) and nitrogen (N_2) as well as the foulsmelling gases methanethiol (CH_4S), hydrogen sulfide (H_2S) and dimethyl sulfide ($(CH_3)_2S$) are also produced in slightly smaller quantities. The short-chain fatty acids include acetate, butyrate and propionate, which in some cases also lead to an odor problem.

Are There Extra-Intestinal Fodmap Effects?

Most of the known effects by FODMAPs arise directly in the colon due to fermentation and its end-products. These end-products cause changes directly in the colon, which in turn lead to symptoms. There are, however, indications that individual FODMAPs also cause other effects in our body, at sites distant from the colon.

In patients with irritable bowel syndrome and fructose malabsorption or lactose intolerance, it was observed that a concurrent mild depression was significantly improved by a fructose or lactose-free diet. It remains unclear, however, whether this depression is caused by fructose malabsorption or lactose intolerance, that is to say that it is directly connected with the disease, or whether it is caused by long-term symptoms, over the years, i.e. appearing secondary to the underlying disease.

Significantly better established is the link between the uptake of fructo-oligosaccharides belonging to FODMAPs and the development of heartburn. Fructo-oligosaccharides can aggravate the reflux of the gastric contents and gastric acid into the esophagus, thereby causing heartburn.

How Do Intestinal Gases Cause Discomfort?

Fermentation of FODMAPs produces gases in large quantities. These gases cause symptoms such as bloating, flatulence and abdominal pain. The precise mechanism of how these gases cause intestinal symptoms is well-established. Various studies have shown that gasses that had been delivered into the intestinal lumen under experimental conditions triggered flatulence and abdominal pain. The severity of the measurable symptoms strongly depends on the amount of intestinal gas. The more intestinal gas and fluid are found in the small and large intestine, the more the intestine is expanded and inflated from the inside, which in turn clinically manifests itself in bloating, flatulence, abdominal pain and loose stools. Additionally, the frequency of bowel movements is higher with increased intestinal contents: on the one hand because more stool volume is produced when digesting high-FODMAP foodstuff, and on the other hand because the increased intestinal filling stimulates intestinal activity, resulting in a more frequent urge to defecate and in thus in more frequent defecation. The currently only unresolved aspect on

FODMAP is how an excess of FODMAPs leads to constipation and hard stools in a small sub-group of people. Irrespective of the lack of an explanation for this, patients with hard stools and constipation also benefit from a lowFODMAP diet.

Besides abdominal pain, many patients also report a bloating sensation, and in some patients meteorism and abdominal distension is indeed objectively recognized by an increase in abdominal circumference. This effect of intestinal gases on the development of symptoms is not detectable solely in patients with IBS, i.e. those with already existing problems, but also in persons without IBS. The only thing that sets them apart is the stimulus threshold, which makes a certain amount of intestinal gas perceived (sometimes painful).

This mechanism of intestinal gases triggering symptoms is particularly clearly established for intestinal gas in the colon and the distal third of the small intestine. However, gases are not the only thing that causes an expansion of the intestine from the inside; distension caused by solid or liquid components in the intestinal lumen may also cause symptoms. This is of high relevance for FODMAPs since bacterial fermentation of the FODMAPs leads to the formation of other bacterial degradation products in addition to gases. These bacterial degradation products cause fluid to flow into the intestinal tract, thereby increasing the liquid and solid intestinal contents. Both contribute to an increased filling of the intestine in addition to the filling by intestinal gases, and intensifies the symptoms. In summary, FODMAPs lead to symptoms or worsening of symptoms through various degradation products. Without a doubt, our intestine is designed for the absorption of gases, fluids and food components from it into the body. However, if our diet is too high in FODMAPs, intestinal gases are produced too quickly and in too large quantity. In turn, too much water is bound in the intestine, in particular due to the short-chain FODMAPs and their degradation products. Since our bodies can no longer compensate for this, the unpleasant symptoms arise. The data from scientific studies are unequivocal and speak for the FODMAP diet. Fewer FODMAPs cause less intestinal gases and less intestinal contents, in turn causing fewer digestive problems.

Visceral Hypersensitivity

Visceral hypersensitivity, also termed the sensitive gut, is highly prevalent in all functional bowel disorders, including irritable bowel syndrome. However, tests for this condition are not offered in daily clinical practice because the derived information would not contribute to any therapeutic decisions, meaning that the patients would not benefit from such tests. Sometimes hypersensitivity tests are carried out in scientific studies. The testing principle is very simple. A balloon is first inserted into the rectum and then gradually inflated. The filling level at which the patient perceives the balloon is called the perception threshold. When the balloon is further inflated, the patient starts to feel pain, which is called the pain threshold. These thresholds are measurable in every patient, and they tend to be shifted in patients with irritable bowel syndrome. Patients with IBS perceive the balloon sooner and the distension is perceived sooner as painful. This is an uncomplicated test that simply and figuratively describes what leads to abdominal pain and other symptoms in patients with irritable bowel syndrome.

! Patients with irritable bowel syndrome have a more sensitive intestinal tract, rendering them more perceptive to pain.

The origin of the hypersensitivity of the intestine has not been clarified yet. In the case of irritable bowel syndrome, a variety of causes are considered possible, including hereditary factors, environmental influences and, last but not least, the intestinal flora. Unfortunately, there is as yet no adequate answer to the question as to why visceral hypersensitivity occurs. But the test principle helps us understand another issue. The test balloon is nothing but a substitute for intestinal gases. It is the intestinal gas filling that leads to paresthesia and pain in patients with a sensitive bowel or IBS. This explains why the same amount of intestinal gas does not cause any discomfort in a healthy person but in a person with IBS.

Activity Of Intestinal Muscles And Transport Velocity

Another point is important in the development of symptoms due to FODMAPs. It is very well known that in patients with IBS, the intestinal wall muscles respond to distension stimuli with increased muscle activity, that is to say, stronger muscle contractions. This leads to abdominal cramps and an increased urge to defecate. For this reason, increased intestinal gases, as they occur after FODMAP consumption, cause abdominal cramping and frequent bowel movements.

Changes In The Intestinal Flora

Several clinical studies have shown that the composition of the intestinal flora in patients with irritable bowel syndrome is significantly altered in comparison to the flora of an unaffected person. However, we do not yet know enough about the "normal" composition of the intestinal flora; hence, the changes in the intestinal flora in patients with IBS cannot be classified. For the same reason, it is also not clear what bacteria are associated with what changes, which kind of bacteria are involved in the development of the symptoms, and what do the detected changes in the intestinal flora in patients with irritable bowel syndrome mean. However, it is conceivable that some bacteria ferment FODMAPs more potently than others; the only thing missing is the evidence that this is the case in patients with irritable bowel syndrome.

! Patients with IBS display an altered intestinal flora as compared with healthy people. Hence, it is conceivable that certain bacteria handle FODMAPs better than others.

It is interesting that the composition of our intestinal flora changes depending on whether we eat a high or low-FODMAP diet. A low-FODMAP diet leads to a reduced presence of various bacteria from the group of Clostridia. Some groups of Clostridia species are very pathogenic and spoil or poison food; hence, it is conceivable that the changes in the intestinal flora of persons on a low-FODMAP diet contribute to the improvement of the digestive problems.

Are The Fodmap Effects Detectable?

Yes, for each and every step in the FODMAP hypothesis, there is strong evidence reflected in human studies. It has been shown that FODMAPs are actually poorly (or not at all) absorbed from the small intestine into the body's circulation and directly enter the colon, where they are fermented by resident bacteria. It has also been demonstrated that this fermentation leads to an increase in the stool volume, in particular by an increase of the liquid components, and that abundant intestinal gas is formed. For individual FODMAPs such as fructose, sorbitol, lactose and fructo-oligosaccharides it has been demonstrated that they can cause symptoms in healthy individuals when they are present in high quantities, while in patients with IBS they can cause symptoms even in much smaller quantities. Numerous clinical studies have also revealed that the effects of the individual FODMAPs are synergistically augmented when ingested together, as is customary in our mixed diet.

Lactulose, The Synthetic Fodmap

Lactulose is an artificial double-sugar consisting of fructose and galactose. In the intestine, lactulose cannot be split into the individual sugars; hence, lactulose cannot be absorbed in the intestine. There are no natural sources of lactulose. Strictly speaking, lactulose is a synthetically produced FODMAP. The actual use of lactulose is rather interesting. It is used as a laxative and characterized in particular by a very good water-binding capacity in the intestine. Thus, lactulose has a laxative effect and causes the stool to soften. Like the other FODMAPs, lactulose also leads to the formation of intestinal gases by fermentation in the colon. For this reason, flatulence is often reported as a side effect when lactulose is taken, in addition to the mentioned laxative effect and looser stools.

In essence, the effects of the laxative lactulose are the best proof of the FODMAP theory.

Chapter 3: Who Benefits From A Low-Fodmap Diet?

The FODMAP concept is very new and has not yet been studied in many diseases. The low-FODMAP diet has been thoroughly studied in patients with irritable bowel syndrome, and in those with bloating and diarrhea. Patients with other diseases like inflammatory bowel disease or food intolerances benefit too, but the current study quality is not yet as good as it is for irritable bowel syndrome. The text below describes the illnesses and symptoms in which a low-FODMAP diet is promising according to our present knowledge.

For whom is a low-FODMAP diet suitable?

Definitely beneficial, investigated in clinical studies:
- Irritable bowel syndrome in children and adults
- Inflammatory bowel disease such as Crohn's disease and ulcerative colitis with

symptoms despite well-controlled intestinal inflammation
- Wheat sensitivity (wheat intolerance)
- Patients who suffer from diarrhea or other symptoms in the hospital

Beneficial, not yet investigated in clinical studies:
- FODMAP intolerance
- Non-specific gastrointestinal symptoms (boating, abdominal pain, diarrhea)
- Fructose malabsorption with an inadequate response to a fructose-reduced diet
- Lactose intolerance with an inadequate response to a lactose-free diet
- Patients in whom colon has been removed and who often have loose or watery stools

Which Diseases Cause Digestive Complaints?

A variety of diseases are associated with digestive problems and gastrointestinal symptoms. This guide is not a substitute for seeing a doctor, and it is important to consult a doctor first in order to prevent serious illness. Often, however, no explanatory causes are found for digestive complaints, and the diagnosis of irritable bowel syndrome is made. In these cases, a low-FODMAP diet is promising. Whether a low-FODMAP diet is promising in cases of digestive problems caused by a diverticular disease of the colon has not yet been established in studies, but when flatulence and loose stools are the chief complaint, it is definitely well worth a try.

Irritable bowel syndrome

Irritable bowel syndrome is a common disease. The patients report bloating, flatulence, abdominal pain and changes in bowel movements. The stool can be too loose, sometimes even watery, or too firm, and defecation may be too frequent or infrequent. These symptoms and changes in bowel movements do not always occur, but rather they can occur only on individual days. It is also not uncommon for the symptoms to appear intermittently or alternately. The causes of irritable bowel syndrome are not fully understood. In addition to a hereditary component, gastrointestinal infections, environmental factors and nutritional factors also play a role. The interplay of all these factors leads to a markedly inconsistent disease pattern. For this reason, the affected persons often do not know for years what is wrong with them. As a result, they see different specialists and subject themselves to a variety of examinations, sometimes for several years, before the right diagnosis is made. The diagnosis of irritable bowel syndrome is made when the above-mentioned digestive complaints occur regularly and limit the quality of life. The physician orders examinations to rule out other diseases, which could explain the symptoms. Depending on the main symptom, different forms of progression are distinguished. They include IBS with diarrhea, IBS with constipation, IBS with abdominal pain, IBS with bloating, and IBS with alternating symptoms. It is important to note that despite the designation according to the main symptom, other digestive symptoms can occur simultaneously. Various forms of irritable bowel syndrome depending on clinical course:

- IBS with diarrhea
- IBS with constipation
- IBS with abdominal pain
- IBS with bloating
- IBS with alternating symptoms

Treatment of irritable bowel syndrome can be achieved by a variety of measures. In addition to drugs, alternative medicine measures and the low-FODMAP diet are also promising.

Fructose malabsorption and symptoms despite a diet low in fructose As mentioned earlier in this guide, fructose malabsorption is an independent disease that can be conclusively diagnosed with a breath test. The treatment includes a diet low in fructose, while a low-FODMAP diet is not necessary in this disease entity. However, some patients with fructose intolerance continue to show signs of indigestion despite a diet low in fructose.

! Fructose malabsorption and irritable bowel syndrome may occur simultaneously as well.

This may be due to the fact that fructose malabsorption and IBS are simultaneously present, which occurs more often than one would imagine. Both diseases are common and can therefore occur concurrently. In such a case, it is worthwhile to add a lowFODMAP diet to the low-fructose diet. That said, however, such a "trial" should not be performed for longer than 6-8 weeks, and a continuation of the FODMAP diet is recommended only if you feel that your symptoms are improving significantly.

Lactose intolerance and symptoms despite a diet low in lactose

Lactose intolerance is diagnosed with special breath tests, as described above for fructose malabsorption. Once lactose intolerance has been conclusively diagnosed, the therapy consists of a lactose-free or at least a lactose-reduced diet. In most patients this leads to a good control of symptoms. In some cases, however, digestive problems persist despite the lactose-free diet. In such a situation, the low-FODMAP diet can be tried. The FODMAP diet should first be maintained for 6-8 weeks. If the symptoms improve, it can be continued. If not, the diet should be discontinued.

Celiac   disease
Celiac disease is an autoimmune disease characterized by an immune reaction against gluten, leading to inflammation of the small intestine and subsequently to symptoms such as bloating and diarrhea. In short, when a patient presents with bloating and diarrhea, celiac disease should be considered.
Gluten is a protein found in wheat, rye and barley. Celiac disease is treated with a glutenfree diet. This gluten-free diet, however, clearly differs from the low-FODMAP diet. It is not necessary to eat gluten-free in the context of a low-FODMAP diet, and a strictly gluten-free diet is not recommended unless celiac disease has been unequivocally diagnosed.
Celiac disease is distinguished from wheat allergy and wheat sensitivity using tissue studies of the small intestine and blood tests detecting antibodies against gluten (tissue transglutaminase antibodies). These antibodies prove the existence of celiac disease. Since celiac disease is not directed against wheat, but rather against gluten, the necessary diet is a gluten-free diet, i.e. wheat, rye, and barley-free.
If you have celiac disease, the low-FODMAP diet is not suitable for you. If, however, you still experience digestive problems despite a strictly gluten-free diet, and your doctor cannot find any other cause that

explains your symptoms, you may find it helpful to try a low-FODMAP diet as well.

Wheat allergy and wheat (gluten) sensitivity
There are two disease presentations that are very similar to celiac disease, namely wheat allergy and wheat sensitivity, also called wheat intolerance, which are often confused. The accurate medical term for wheat sensitivity is actually "non-celiac wheat (gluten) sensitivity". These diseases are confused very frequently since they are characterized by very similar symptoms, they are accompanied by very similar intolerances, namely the intolerance to wheat, and they are treated with very similar measures, namely wheat-free diets. Nevertheless, they are different diseases.

Celiac disease can be distinguished very well from wheat allergy and wheat (gluten) sensitivity. Wheat allergy is also characterized by the formation of antibodies in the body. However, these antibodies are not directed against gluten, but rather against other wheat proteins such as gliadins and thioredoxins. This disease is a real allergy. However, not all of these antibodies can be detected in clinical laboratory tests. In addition to the digestive problems such as bloating, abdominal cramps, abdominal pain, nausea and diarrhea, wheat allergy may additionally present with allergic symptoms of the skin, lungs, eyes and mouth.

The diagnosis of wheat allergy is sometimes complex because the serum antibodies we know may be absent. Further diagnostic studies, such as gastroscopy, ileoscopy and colonoscopy may contribute a variety of non-specific clues, but they cannot provide a definitive diagnosis. If you have wheat allergy, the lowFODMAP diet is not a suitable diet for you. Wheat (gluten) sensitivity is a disease in which no known antibodies are formed and thus no detection with blood tests is possible. The symptoms of wheat (gluten) sensitivity is more akin to celiac disease. The chief complaint are digestive problems. To make the diagnosis, it is necessary to first exclude celiac disease and wheat allergy. A carefully kept food-symptom-diary can lead to the right direction. On the other hand, many additional complaints are reported in wheat (gluten) sensitivity. Muscle, bone and joint problems as well as headache, fatigue, lassitude and concentration problems have been described. Whether all these symptoms actually belong to wheat sensitivity or whether they are part of a more complex, hitherto not fully understood, disease pattern is currently a subject of heated debate.

! Wheat allergy, wheat (gluten) sensitivity, and celiac disease are frequently confused due to the similar symptoms, but they are actually three separate diseases.

It is not clarified which components of wheat lead to wheat (gluten) sensitivity, that is, to hypersensitivity. The trigger is presumably not gluten; hence, the term gluten sensitivity, which is frequently used, should no longer be used as an umbrella term. The wheat protein amylase trypsin inhibitor (ATI) is currently strongly suspected of triggering the hypersensitivity in wheat sensitivity. The interesting thing about this protein is that it is less present in older wheat varieties than in modern high-performance wheat, i.e. wheat bred with modern methods to bring as high yields as possible. This could be an explanation as to why an increasing number of people suffer from wheat sensitivity.

Differences between celiac disease, wheat allergy, and wheat sensitivity (Gluten sensitivity)

Celiac disease:
Period from food intake to symptoms: Weeks to years
Blood tests: Transglutaminase antibodies
Skin test: No
Inflammation of the small intestine: marked Long-term sequelae: 1:100
Diet: gluten-free

Wheat allergy:
Period from food intake to symptoms: Hours to days
Blood tests: Wheat IgE antibodies (with limitations)

Skin test: Yes
Inflammation of the small intestine: mild (possible)
Long-term sequelae: 1:100 assumed
Diet: wheat-free

Wheat sensitivity (Gluten sensitivity):
Period from food intake to symptoms: Hours to days
Blood tests: none
Skin test: No
Inflammation of the small intestine: Unclear, possibly mild
Long-term sequelae: 1:50 - 1:100 assumed
Diet: low-FODMAP or low-wheat

There is a body of evidence in the literature that FODMAPs can trigger symptoms of wheat sensitivity. Very relevant here is a clinical study involving patients with wheat (gluten) sensitivity, who were treated with a low-FODMAP diet for two weeks. Interestingly, a low-FODMAP diet reduced the symptoms in all patients. The second part of the study is highly interesting as well: After two weeks of the low-FODMAP diet, one group of patients received a bit of gluten added to their diet, while the other group received a lot of gluten. In both groups, symptoms appeared in some patients, but it did not matter whether they received little or much gluten. This implies that gluten is not responsible for the symptoms of wheat sensitivity.

Currently, there are still significant gaps in our understanding of wheat sensitivity. Further research is needed. Some experts even question the existence of this disease. According to the results of the clinical trials, however, instituting a low-FODMAP diet is worth a try in cases of confirmed or suspected wheat sensitivity. A gluten-free diet does not seem to benefit patients with wheat sensitivity, and there is no adequate information on whether a strictly wheat-free diet is effective.

Inflammatory bowel disease: Crohn's disease and ulcerative colitis

Inflammatory bowel disease such as Crohn's disease and ulcerative colitis are characterized by inflammation of the small intestine. In severe cases, they are treated with drugs. In some patients with inflammatory bowel disease, however, digestive problems persist, although the inflammation of the gut responds well to drug treatment which curtails the intestinal inflammation and normalizes inflammatory parameters in the blood. This is then a case of functional intestinal complaints associated with an inflammatory bowel disease.

Such functional intestinal complaints are 2 to 3 times as frequent in patients with a welltreated inflammatory bowel disease as in the normal population. If no other causes are found, it is assumed that these functional complaints correspond to those of irritable bowel syndrome, prompting the same treatment. Therefore, in this case, instituting a lowFODMAP diet is well worth a try. Such an approach is supported by findings in clinical trials in patients with inflammatory bowel disease.

Intestinal surgery

For various medical reasons, it may be necessary to partially or completely remove the colon. As a result of this, digestive discomfort with bloating, abdominal pain, flatulence and loose stools often occur. A low-FODMAP diet is helpful in this case in order to get these symptoms under control or at the very least to achieve a significant relief.

Chapter 4: Understanding Diets

Many patients with digestive problems such as bloating, flatulence, abdominal pain, loose stools or even diarrhea are convinced that the diet is the culprit for their symptoms, or that certain food ingredients are the direct cause of their symptoms. The affected persons observe that the symptoms occur shortly after food intake or that the symptoms occur repeatedly after the intake of certain foods.
Patients often report that after getting up, and during the first hours of the day (in connection with breakfast), they experience increased bowel movements and more frequent loose to watery stools. During the course of the day, bowel movements normalize. The next morning, however, everything starts all over again. However, such observation often has nothing to do with the composition of food. Rather, the culprit are increased gastrointestinal reflexes in a sensitive gut because the activity of the digestive system is usually highest in the morning hours and immediately after a meal, while it decreases during the day and between meals.
Another common observation is that the symptoms occur directly after eating certain foods. This may indicate an intolerance. But here too it should be noted that symptoms that occur directly after food intake are

frequently not caused by an intolerance. Foods that actually cause an intolerance must first pass through the stomach in order to enter the small intestine. Only there do such intolerances lead to symptoms. In essence, it takes a certain time before symptoms appear.

Unraveling intolerances

For these reasons, detecting food intolerances is sometimes a complex task. In the case of a severe intolerance with serious and promptly manifest symptoms, it is somewhat easier to recognize the correlation and to initiate the necessary diagnostic work-up. On the other hand, a mild intolerance with mild symptoms often makes it very difficult to recognize the correlation and to commence the required work-up.

In order to be absolutely certain that a person suffers from a food intolerance, it is helpful to have the patient keep a food-symptom-diary in order to get a better overall picture. In such a diary, all meals, the individual food ingredients, and the exact time of food intake are recorded over a limited period of time, typically four weeks; in addition, it is documented whether the person experienced symptoms or not, and if so which complaints occurred at what time.

If a food intolerance is unequivocally established, a corresponding diet should be followed.

Diets For Irritable Bowel Syndrome

If a patient has irritable bowel syndrome, and food allergy or intolerance has been excluded, the decision as to whether a particular diet should be followed or not, and which one, is not quite so simple. Since irritable bowel syndrome is a disease with many causes and triggers, there has been no standardized diet beneficial to all patients. The medical literature contains a variety of dietary approaches designed to alleviate the symptoms of irritable bowel syndrome or individual symptoms affecting the bowel. Numerous diets are based on the fact that a diet designed to help with food intolerances may also be used to improve symptoms such as bloating or changes in bowel movements in patients with IBS. Although many of these diets follow very clear and rational explanatory models, it is difficult to prove that these dietary changes actually lead to symptom relief. These concepts work in individual cases or in small patient groups. This is why they are occasionally recommended. However, most of these recommendations were not tested in large patient groups. Therefore, no standardized IBS diet has been proposed thus far. This has now fundamentally changed with the advent of a low-FODMAP diet.

The Gradual Path To A Low-Fodmap Diet

If a dietary therapy is to be carried out in symptomatic patients, it is advisable to proceed in three steps. This step-by-step approach is delineated in great detail by the British National Institute for Health and Care Excellence (NICE Institute).

IBS Diet is a three-step process.
If the first step is not helpful, proceed to the second step. However, if the symptoms improve, there is no need to proceed to the next step.
- 1st step: General nutritional recommendations
- 2nd step: Low-FODMAP diet
- 3rd step: Elimination diet

We start with some general nutritional recommendations.
It may be a good idea to keep a food-symptom-diary for a period of four weeks in order to recognize individual food sensitivities and to adjust the dietary plan accordingly. These general recommendations are typically implemented for eight weeks. If an adequate symptom relief is attained, the diet can be continued. However, if these general measures are not sufficient, the next step is to start a diet which omits poorly digestible foods. This is where the low-FODMAP diet comes into play, because the low-FODMAP diet has

been most thoroughly clinically tried and tested for IBS. Hence, it is recommended in this case. According to the results of clinical trials, the low-FODMAP diet will benefit all patients with irritable bowel syndrome, regardless of whether they pass stools that are too loose or too solid. Clinical studies offer concrete evidence for the improvement of bloating, flatulence and abdominal pain.
Most patients report an improvement in stool consistency while on a low-FODMAP diet. Patients with diarrhea have fewer bowel movements and can expect to pass firmer stools. A treatment trial with a low-FODMAP diet should be performed for 6-8 weeks, like any other dietary trial.
Resorting to the third recommendation, which is a strict elimination diet, is justified only in a few isolated cases that fail to respond to a low-FODMAP diet. However, the elimination diet should not be carried out without consulting a doctor or nutritionist, and is therefore beyond the scope of this Guide.

Nutritional recommendations for the symptomatic treatment of bloating, abdominal pain and loose stools

- Eat your meals regularly, typically three main meals and, if necessary, one to two (light) snacks;
- Take enough time to eat your food in a peaceful environment, avoid eating in a rush, or eating while

walking or standing;
- Drink sufficient amounts of fluid, at least 1.5 liters distributed throughout the day, ideally water or tea, and avoid caffeinated drinks;
- Limit the consumption of coffee and black tea to a maximum of 3 cups a day;
- Avoid alcoholic or carbonated drinks;
- Limit the consumption of fresh fruit to a maximum of three servings per day (each with a maximum of 100 g);
- Eat more oats and linseed (1 teaspoon / day) if you suffer from bloating and flatulence;
- Avoid artificial sweeteners if you have diarrhea or loose stools; these are often contained in beverages and low-calorie foods;
- Avoid resistant and retrograded starch.

What Makes The Fodmap Diet Credible?

There are numerous nutritional recommendations that promise relief from bloating, abdominal pain and altered bowel movements. Why should I believe that the lowFODMAP diet is any better? There are several reasons for it.

Initially, a concept was developed for the low-FODMAP diet based on the question of what pathological changes in the bowel cause symptoms. The next step involved identifying those food ingredients that cause changes such as increased intestinal gas, increased abdominal pain or watery stools. All these food ingredients have been summarized under the umbrella term "FODMAP".

Subsequently, the low-FODMAP diet was tested in clinical trials to see whether the symptoms indeed improve. These trials are up-to-date and of high quality. The patients with symptoms were randomized (i.e. assigned randomly) into two groups: one group received a standard Western diet, and the other group a low-FODMAP diet. Patients did not know which diet they were receiving. Such studies enable a dietary concept to be tested without bias. The FODMAP diet has demonstrated its superiority in these studies, and has since been recommended by specialist associations.

! The low-FODMAP diet is based on a scientific concept that was tested and confirmed in various clinical studies.

Are Fodmaps Unhealthy Or Even Dangerous?

The clear-cut answer to this question is "No". FODMAPs are neither unhealthy nor dangerous. FODMAPs are naturally-occurring food ingredients; in some cases they are even added to industrially processed foods. FODMAPs become an issue only when they are ingested in excessive amounts. Our gastrointestinal tract can deal with them to a certain extent. Since FODMAPs are for the most part very poorly digestible, they are not absorbed in the small intestine and enter the colon, where they are digested by the resident bacteria. FODMAPs are literally "fast food" for our gut bacteria. As a rule, FODMAPs are no problem for our bodies - as long as everything works well. Only if too many FODMAPs arrive in the colon, the resident bacteria have too many FODMAPs to digest. Consequently, too many bacterial digestive products overwhelm our intestines. These include intestinal gases. For people with a more robust physique, this turns out to be no problem, the body can handle it. For those with a more sensitive gut, however, the increased intestinal gases are already a problem, and

they readily develop symptoms. In this way, an essentially healthy person can turn into a patient with frequent digestive complaints if his/her diet contains too many FODMAPs. Likewise, a patient with well-controlled digestive symptoms can turn into a patient with uncontrollable, recalcitrant symptoms.
What happens when a healthy person follows a low-FODMAP diet?
Nothing. Since healthy people have no complaints, they cannot improve. The diet is tested on healthy subjects, and a healthy person perceives the changes in the type of food consumed, but that is it.

Is There A Risk Of Nutritional Deficiencies?

No. On the one hand, the low-FODMAP diet only reduces and does not completely eliminate FODMAPs; on the other hand, FODMAPs are not essential food ingredients, which means that a deficiency is expected neither in the healthy nor in patients with symptoms, even if the FODMAP share in their diet is reduced to the very minimum.

How Many Meals A Day Should I Eat?

When on a low-FODMAP diet, you should eat as normally as possible. This also applies to the number of meals eaten. The general nutritional recommendations stipulate three main meals and, if necessary, one or two (light) snacks, ideally consisting of small quantities of fruit. These guidelines should be followed when on a low-FODMAP diet as well. If this is not enough for you, please refer to the FODMAP table to identify foods low in FODMAPs that can serve as additional snacks.

Is The Positive Effect Of The Low-Fodmap Diet Proven?

There are numerous dietary and nutritional suggestions for improving symptoms of irritable bowel syndrome or digestive symptoms of other causes. Some of these recommendations are well-supported by clinical trials, others less well. However, most of the diets are based on traditions or expert opinions and have not been studied in clinical trials, at least not in well-designed trials. This does not mean that all these diets are ineffective, but only that their efficacy is not adequately documented.

The situation regarding evidence is somewhat different for the low-FODMAP diet. This dietary concept was initially proposed by an Australian expert panel as a hypothesis. The hypothesis was essentially based on a variety of nutritional symptom analyses published by various authors and newly interpreted by the said group of experts. Next, this lowFODMAP dietary concept was tested on small patient groups. As it had turned out that the concept works and that a low-FODMAP diet actually offers symptom relief, elaborate clinical trials were initiated involving a large number of patients with irritable bowel syndrome. To date, six clinical trials of highest quality and countless additional clinical trials furnished data on the low-FODMAP diet.

In the largest study, the patients received either a low-FODMAP diet or a normal diet for three weeks. The patients were again randomized (i.e. randomly assigned) to a dietary plan. After three weeks of therapy, the patients on one diet received the other diet for three weeks afterwards. During the entire study period, symptoms such as abdominal pain, abdominal cramps, bloating and diarrhea were recorded. The remarkable thing about this large clinical study was that neither the patients nor their study doctors knew whether the patients were in the low-FODMAP or the normal diet group at any point in time. In medicine, such studies are called double-blind studies because no one knows -neither the doctor nor the patient -- which therapy a particular patient is receiving. It is precisely this design that makes double-blind studies so meaningful, since the study results cannot be influenced consciously or unconsciously in such a study. To date (year 2016), the concept of a low-

FODMAP diet has been studied in countless studies in many countries around the world. In doing so, the FODMAP diet was adapted to the local diet and, in particular, locally different serving sizes. Thus, the concept can be examined in studies in very different countries.

Resistant Starch, Retrograded Starch: What Are They?

Resistant starch is starch that cannot be digested by the digestive enzymes in the small intestine, and therefore enters the colon where it can cause symptoms after conversion by the resident bacteria. High quantities of resistant starch are found, for example, in green bananas and in certain corn varieties.
Retrograded starch is starch that becomes indigestible by heating and subsequent cooling. Retrograded starch is found particularly after heating foods rich in starch such as potatoes and cereal products, as well as in industrially processed foods. We do not yet know the content of resistant starch in most foods. The generation of resistant starch is very variable and depends on the food, on the type of preparation, duration and temperature, as well as on many other circumstances.

What You Should Know About Fiber

A frequent recommendation in the past was that the amount of dietary fiber should be increased in patients with irritable bowel syndrome. However, this recommendation does not work for all affected persons since many dietary fibers arrive in the colon in an undigested form, and are decomposed by resident bacteria. This applies in particular to the water-insoluble plant fiber which we take in with fruits, vegetables, cereals and bran. During bacterial decomposition, intestinal gases are generated, and these intestinal gases cause symptoms. Therefore, dietary fiber, especially the water-insoluble dietary fiber, often leads to a paradoxical, counterproductive effect in patients with digestive complaints by making their symptoms stronger rather than weaker.

Water-soluble fiber, such as psyllium and linseed, bind water in the intestine and thus act as stool-regulating agents, their effects best unfolded in the granulated, crushed or ground form.

The current state-of-the-art recommendation is that the diet should be supplemented with water-soluble dietary fibers in patients with symptoms of irritable bowel syndrome. In the intestine, the water-soluble dietary fibers bind abundant water and lead to better stool consistency, regular bowel movements, and thus symptom relief. Water-soluble fibers are less potently decomposed by bacteria in the colon, thereby generating less additional intestinal gas. Therefore, water-soluble dietary fibers such as psyllium or psyllium husks are considered stool-regulating products.

Psyllium products which are available in pharmacies and health food stores in various forms are produced from the Indian plantain. Psyllium husks can bind up to 50 times their weight of water in the intestine. The effect of granulated or ground psyllium is better than the effect of untreated one. In addition to psyllium, oat is also rich in water-soluble fiber and is suitable for fiber fortification and additional water binding. Linseed is also rich in water-soluble fiber, but should only be crushed or best ground, since it is otherwise ineffective and appears undigested in the stool.

The influence of the composition of the intestinal flora on the digestion of dietary fiber is not clear. What we know, however, is that patients with digestive problems produce more intestinal gases from dietary fiber, report increased flatulence, have more severe abdominal pain, and a different composition of the intestinal flora than patients without digestive problems. Although it is still too early to name the bacteria responsible for increased intestinal gas production, bacteria with fun names like Bacillus uniformis, Bilophila wadsworthia and Parabacteroides distasonis are among the suspects.

Chapter 5: The First Step Is Always The Hardest

In the previous chapters, you learned about the basics of the low-FODMAP diet. Now let's implement this knowledge. It is nearly impossible to obtain information on each food in detail, and to measure the content of the individual FODMAPs in these foods. This is not necessary either. As the name implies, the low-FODMAP diet is not about eating no FODMAPs at all because this is not possible, but rather, it is about identifying foods low in FODMAPs and avoiding foods that are high in FODMAPs. Since various FODMAPs are contained in different quantities in different foodstuffs, it is the overall assessment of the individual foodstuffs that counts. The content of various FODMAPs is included in this overall assessment; subsequently, the food is classified as low or high in FODMAPs. A lemon, for example, which contains moderate amounts of fructose and traces of polyols, is classified as low in FODMAPs overall, since it contains only a low share from the other FODMAP groups. The following table shows the assessment of FODMAP content of individual foods.

These are examples of FODMAP content evaluation of individual foods, and how the overall assessment is achieved:

Rice: fructose: traces; lactose: traces; oligosaccharides: none; polyols: none overall assessment: low in FODMAPs

Pear: fructose: much; lactose: none; oligosaccharides: none; polyols: much overall assessment: high in FODMAPs

Lemon: fructose: moderate; lactose: none; oligosaccharides: traces; polyols: traces overall assessment: low in FODMAPs

Cherries: fructose: much; lactose: none; oligosaccharides: traces; polyols: traces overall assessment: high in FODMAPs

Strawberries: fructose: moderate; lactose: none; oligosaccharides: traces; polyols: moderate overall assessment: low in FODMAPs

FODMAP content of individual foods, and how the overall assessment is arrived at

	Fructose	Lactose	Oligo-saccharides	Polyols	Overall assessment
Rice	traces	traces	none	none	low in FODMAPs
Pear	much	none	none	much	high in FODMAPs
Lemon	moderate	none	traces	traces	low in FODMAPs
Cherries	much	none	traces	traces	high in FODMAPs
Strawberries	moderate	none	traces	moderate	low in FODMAPs

In order to be able to create a successful low-FODMAP diet for yourself, please refer to the tables with listing of foods high in FODMAPs and foods low in FODMAPs in this book. These must be either selected or avoided. To simplify your grocery shopping, we have reprinted these tables in the cover of this book for you to copy and take along.

! Please note that the tables are only an aid providing a rough guidance on food assessment.
! The size of the servings also plays a role in tolerability since you take in more FODMAPs with a larger serving.

! For example, you may be able to eat a very small amount of a food high in FODMAPs without experiencing symptoms, but you will experience discomfort when eating a very large quantity of a food that is actually classified as low in FODMAPs.

How Can I Reduce Fodmaps In My Diet?

The FODMAP content depends on where you live, your culture and the local characteristics of your diet. Our Western lifestyle is characterized by a diet that is particularly rich in fructose, fructans and polyols. Initially, the foods high in FODMAPs should be avoided, but later they can be consumed again in small quantities. On the other hand, you can mix and match foods low in FODMAPs at will to create your diet. If you have decided to try the low-FODMAP diet, strongly consider doing grocery shopping yourself, preparing your own meals, and preparing them from as few different foods as possible. This will simplify your low-FODMAP diet.

Foods that contain lots of FODMAPs and whose consumption should be reduced

Fruits, high in FODMAP: Apple, Apricot, Avocado, Pear, Blackberries, Figs, Pomegranate, Grapefruit, Guave, unripe, Currant, Kaki (persimmons), Cherries, Lychees, Mango, Mirabelle, Nashi pear, Nectarine, Peach, Plums, Prune, Watermelon, Sugar banana, ripe Canned fruits, Cocoa water, Fruit juices, Dried fruits

Vegetables and legumes, high in FODMAP: Artichoke, Cauliflower, Beans (except green beans), Peas, Green onion (white part), Garlic, Cabbage, Leek (white part), Lentils, Mushrooms, Beetroot, Shallot, Black salsify, Soybeans, Asparagus, Sweet potato, Girasole, Savoy, Sweet peas, Sweet corn, Onion

Cereals and grain products, high in FODMAP: Bread, cereals, pastries, semolina, flakes, pasta, flour, etc. from: amaranth, barley, unripe spelt grain, rye, triticale, wheat, Lupin flour Bulgur, Couscous, Wheat germ

Dairy products and milk substitutes, high in FODMAP:

Butter milk, Cream cheese, Yogurt, Coffee cream, Creamer, Kefir , Condensed milk, Ice milk, Milk powder , Whey , Whey powder, Quark / Curd, Cream, Sour cream, Heavy sour cream, Soy milk * (from soybeans) , Tsatsiki, Cheese, Farmer cheese, Halloumi, Mascarpone, Whey cheese
*FODMAP content varies, depending on the processing

Other foods, high in FODMAP:
Sweeteners: Maple sirup, Fructose sirup, Honey, Corn sirup, Sugar substitutes (ending with -it or -ol)
Chocolate: Milk chocolate, White chocolate, Carob chocolate
Nuts: Cashew nuts, Pistachios
Alcohol, drinks: Beer (more than one glass), Liqueur, Port wine, Rum, Sherry, Wine, sparkling wine (semi-dry; sweet)
Plant protein: Vegetable protein, Silken tofu

Foods that contain few FODMAPs and are suitable for a low-FODMAP diet (SS)=Small serving; *FODMAP content varies depending on the preparation

Fruits, low in FODMAP
Pineapple, Banana, Blueberries, Cantaloupe melon, Clementine, Pitaya, Durian, Strawberries, Galia melon, Guave, ripe, Raspberries, Prickly pear, Carambola, Chestnuts, Kiwi, Kumquat, Lime, Tangerine, Maracuja, Sweet chestnuts, Net melon, Orange, Papaya, Rhubarb, Starfruit, Grapes, Lemon, Muskmelon

Vegetables and legumes, low in FODMAP:
Alfalfa, Eggplant, Broccoli (ss), Chicorée salad, Chillies, Chinese cabbage, Fennel, Green onion (green part), Green beans, Cucumber, Hokkaido, Ginger, Carrot, Potato, Kohlrabi, Chickpeas * (ss), Celeriac (ss), Leek (green part), Corn * (ss), Maniok (ss), Chard , Okra, Olives, Pepper, Parsnip, Radishes, Radish, Brussel sprout (ss), Red cabbage, Salad/lettuce, Chives, Soybean sprouts, Spaghetti squash, Spinach, Celery (ss), Tomato, White cabbage, Zucchini

Cereals and grain products, low in FODMAP:
Bread, cereals, pastries, semolina, flakes, pasta, flour, etc. made from: Buckwheat, spelt flour*, oats*, millet, corn (polenta), quinoa, rice, tapioca

Potato starch, Popcorn, Cornflakes (ss), Potato chips (ss), Corn chips (ss)

Dairy products and milk substitutes, low in FODMAP:
Lactose-free milk, Lactose-free dairy products, Butter, Margarine (Oleo), Coconut milk,, Soy milk* (from soy protein)
Cheese: Mountain cheese, Brie, Mild, full-flat cheese, Camembert, Cheddar, Chester, Edamer, Emmentaler, Feta, Gorgonzola, Gouda, Hard cheese, Harzer cheese, Mozzarella, Parmesan, Pecorino, Raclette, Ricotta, Tilsiter

Other foods, low in FODMAP:
Sweeteners: Maple sirup, Aspartam, Stevia, Sugar (white, brown), Sugar sirup **Chocolate:** Dark chocolate
Nuts and Seeds: Always fewer than 15 pieces of: hazelnuts, macadamia, almonds, Brazil nuts, pecan, walnuts; **Always less than 15 g of:**, chia seeds, peanuts, pumpkin seeds, sesame seeds, sunflower seeds
Alcohol, drinks: Beer (not more than 1 glass), Wine (dry)
Meat and plant protein: Eggs, fish and meat, Seafood, Tofu (solid, without additions), Tempeh
Oils and sauces: Vinegar, Vegetable oils, Mustard, Soy sauce

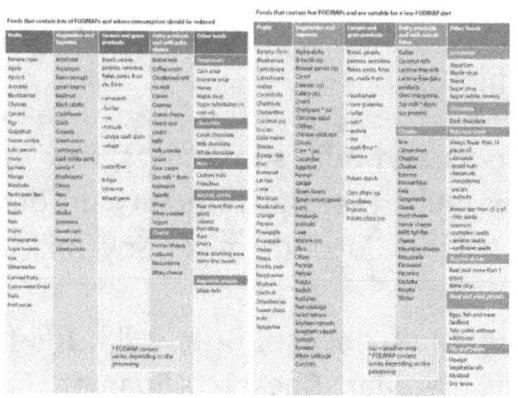

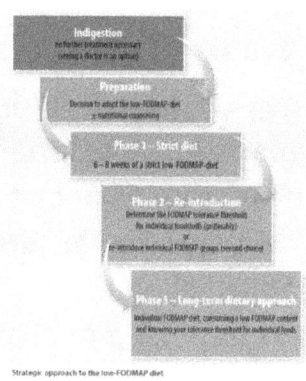

Strategic approach to the low-FODMAP diet

Ready-made meals, ready-to-serve sauces and the like are best avoided because their FODMAP content is difficult to control. Since it is not possible to know the FODMAP content especially of fresh fruits and vegetables, it is a good idea to take along a copy of the FODMAP lists when grocery shopping in order to be able to distinguish foods that are low in FODMAPs from those that are high in FODMAPs.

Low-FODMAP diet, phase 1: Strictly low in FODMAPs
The first phase of the low-FODMAP diet lasts 6 to 8 weeks. At this time, you should strictly adhere to your low-FODMAP diet in order to obtain maximum therapeutic success. Choose only foods low in FODMAPs from the food tables, and prepare your own meals. As you can see from the tables, there are plenty of foods available, you need not worry about having to eat a monotonous diet...

! The FODMAP diet is not a very restrictive one. Even in the strict phase 1, nutritional deficiencies are not expected.

To make phase 1 of the FODMAP diet as easy on yourself as possible, in this book you will find a replacement table. At this stage, you should select only foods listed in the green table and strictly avoid those in the red table. In the second part of this book, you will find some recipes that will help you get started with your low-FODMAP diet. You will find recipe suggestions for the main meals - breakfast, lunch and dinner. You will also find suggestions for starters and desserts. Since the topic of bread requires a lot of attention, you will also find recipes for making your own bread and for the bread baking machine.

! The strict phase 1 of the low-FODMAP diet is not a life-long diet.

In the first 6-8 weeks, it is about getting rid of the digestive problems and getting to know the maximum possible success. During this phase you will also develop greater awareness of food and ways to prepare it. This more conscious approach often adds to a more positive attitude towards life. When you have successfully mastered this period, you will proceed to Diet Phase 2.

! The strict Phase 1 lasts only 6 to 8 weeks . You can look forward to a more liberal

Phase 2.
Replacement tables: High-FODMAP foods are replaced by low-FODMAP ones (selection)

Fruit
Foods high in FODMAPs ... Apple, apricot, avocado, pear, blackberries, grapefruit, currants, cherries, lychees, mango, Nashi pear, nectarine, persimmon, peach, plums, watermelon, prune
replaced by alternatives low in FODMAPs... Pineapple, banana, blueberries, clementine, strawberries, raspberries, honeymelon, kiwi, lime, tangerine,

maracuja, net melon, orange, papaya, rhubarb, grapes, lemon

Vegetables and legumes
Foods high in FODMAPs ... Artichoke, cauliflower, beans (all except green string beans), peas, green onion (white part), garlic, cabbage, leek (white part), lentils, mushrooms, beetroot, soybeans, asparagus, sweet potato, savoy cabbage, sugar peas, sweetcorn, onion **replaced by alternatives low in FODMAPs...** Alfalfa, eggplant, broccoli (small serving), chicory lettuce, chinese cabbage, fennel, green onion (green part), green string beans, cucumber, Hokkaido pumpkin, ginger, carrot, potato, kohlrabi, chickpeas (small serving, soak and pour off water), leeks (green part), chard, okra, olives, peppers, parsnips, radish, Brussel sprouts (small serving), lettuce, chives, soy sprouts, spinach, celery (small serving), tomato, white cabbage, zucchini

Flour, grains
Foods high in FODMAPs ... Wheat products (wheat semolina, wheat germ, wheat bran, bulgur, couscous), barley, rye, triticale, amaranth and lupine **replaced by alternatives low in FODMAPs...** Products made of buckwheat, oats, millet, corn, quinoa, rice, tapioca, potato flour (FODMAP content may vary depending on processing).

Dairy products
Foods high in FODMAPs ... Cream cheese, yogurt, condensed milk, mascarpone, milk powder, milk ice cream, cream, sour cream
replaced by alternatives low in FODMAPs... Lactose-free milk, lactose-free dairy products, Brie, Camembert, Cheddar, Feta, hard cheese, mozzarella, Parmesan

Sweetening agents
Foods high in FODMAPs ... Agave sirup, fructose sirup, honey, corn sirup, sugar substitutes ending in -it or ol (mannitol, sorbitol, maltitol, xylitol)
replaced by alternatives low in FODMAPs... Maple sirup, aspartame, rice sirup, stevia, sugar (white, brown), sugar sirup

Nuts and seeds
Foods high in FODMAPs ... **Cashew nuts, pistachios** replaced by alternatives low in FODMAPs... **All other nuts and seeds in small quantities**

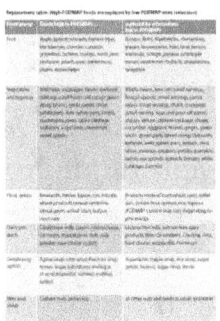

FODMAP Diet Phase 2: Re-introduction of foods

In the first few weeks, you learned how your digestive problems improve if you follow an optimal low-FODMAP diet. However, the long-term goal is not to permanently adhere to a strict low-FODMAP diet. Phase 2 of the diet is about re-introducing a wider variety of possible foods to make your diet richer and more diverse. This can be accomplished in a variety of ways.

! Design your own FODMAP diet. The more care you take in Phase 2 when reintroducing different food groups/foods, the more you will benefit from your lowFODMAP diet in the long run.

Reintroducing individual foods

One way is to slowly re-introduce individual foods into the diet and gradually increase the amount of these foods. These steps should proceed slowly, each step ideally takes 3-4 days, since the intestine is a rather inert organ and it can take 3-4 days from food intake to the emergence of symptoms. This will tell you the maximum amount of a foodstuff high in FODMAPs that you still tolerate well enough without developing digestive symptoms. It is of utmost importance to investigate each foodstuff separately. For any food that is high in FODMAPs, and which you cannot do without, you can learn what amount your body will tolerate without digestive discomfort. These tolerability thresholds are very different. Your goal should be to figure out your personal threshold. If you find that some foods cause digestive problems in very small amounts already, you should remove them from your diet for good.

Reintroducing FODMAP categories
It is up to you to decide whether you want to start reintroducing individual foods or different FODMAP categories. The introduction of individual foodstuffs is easier, so this procedure is recommended.
If you want to test your tolerability of FODMAP groups, the following foods are suitable for a tolerance test for the various FODMAP groups.

! This testing is best accomplished if you have a written plan to follow. ! Be sure to test only individual foods or FODMAP groups, otherwise you may loose track and can no longer correctly assign symptoms or complaints.

Fructose tolerance is tested using two spoonfuls of honey, which is very high in fructose, or alternatively, three apples. A glass of whole milk is suitable for testing lactose tolerance. To test your fructane tolerance, use an onion or one or two cloves of garlic. Galactan tolerance is tested with a lentil dish. Testing polyol tolerability is somewhat more difficult, since polyols and fructose occur together in most natural products. A test with five pieces of sorbitol and mannitol-containing chewing gum appears suitable.

FODMAP Diet Phase 3 - The long-term dietary approach

Once Phase 2 is completed, you begin your personal diet. You know those foods high in FODMAPs that you can tolerate and also those that you cannot tolerate. You know your tolerance threshold for individual high-FODMAP foods. You will find that you hardly tolerate some high-FODMAP foods even in very small quantities. Some patients realize at the end of Phase 2 that they can enjoy an almost normal diet and that they cannot tolerate only isolated high-FODMAP foods. Others, on the other hand, realize that they do not tolerate polyols at all, but that they are more or less OK with all other FODMAPs. The goal is to find your individual, diverse and balanced diet, that enables you to stay permanently symptom-free. In general, you should treat all foods whose FODMAP content you do not know, as well as all industrially processed foods that do not provide sufficient information on the ingredients, as foods high in FODMAPs. You will probably be able to evaluate industrially processed mixed foods in the long term, and to gradually reintroduce them into your diet, if this is still something you want to do.

! Hands off food whose FODMAP content you do not know and cannot assess!!
You will most likely slide back into a high-FODMAP diet when you create your individual diet. This is not uncommon, there are ups and downs in our lives. Simply reexamine your diet to identify dietary errors, and adjust it.

If The Low-Fodmap Diet Does Not Help

In some cases, the low-FODMAP diet brings no improvement or only a partial improvement of the digestive problems. There are various reasons for this. One possible reason is that an individual high-FODMAP foodstuff slipped into your diet. In order to get to the bottom of this, again carefully review the FODMAP food list to identify any such dietary errors and adjust the diet accordingly.
Another reason why the low-FODMAP diet does not help may be that another disorder or intolerance is

responsible for your digestive problems, such as intolerance to food additives such as gluten or other naturally occurring food chemicals such as amygdalin in fruit cores, glycoalkaloids such as solanine in potatoes, lectins in beans, cucurbitacins in zucchini and oxalic acid in rhubarb leaves. Intolerances to these substances are, however, rare.

What About Cheese?

Individual cheese varieties contain FODMAPs in different quantities. The essential FODMAP in cheese is lactose. Lactose contained in milk is decomposed during cheese production by the enzyme lactase, which is mostly derived from bacteria during the production of cheese. Therefore, the FODMAP/lactose content in cheese varieties with a long aging time is lower than in cheese varieties with a little to no aging time. Cheese varieties with a long aging time such as hard cheese, feta cheese, Camembert and Brie, are well-suited for a low-FODMAP diet. Cheese varieties with a short aging time such as cream cheese and cottage cheese are high in FODMAPs because of their high lactose content, and therefore not very suitable.
 You should know the lactose content of the different types of cheese in order to assess their FODMAP content. Refer to the following table for the lactose

content of different types of cheese. In the upper half of the table you can find the most suitable cheese varieties (low in lactose), while in the lower half of the table you will find unsuitable types of cheese (high in lactose). Since the lactose content in various products can fluctuate, the values in the table are only a rough guide.

What About Other Dairy Products?

It is important to know the lactose content of other dairy products as well. Different dairy products contain lactose in different amounts. In the upper part of the table you will find dairy products with a low lactose content, and in the lower part products with a high lactose content. Since the lactose content in the various products can fluctuate, the values in this table are also merely a rough guide.

Lactose content in cheese in g/100 g Low lactose content
Mountain cheese < 0.1
Brie 0.1–0.2
Mild, full-fat cheese < 0.1–1
Camembert 0.1–0.2
Chester < 0.1
Edamer < 0.1
Emmentaler < 0.1

Feta 0.5
Gouda < 0.1
Harzer cheese < 0.1
Mozzarella < 0,1
Parmesan < 0.1
Raclette < 0.1
Ricotta 0.3
Tilsiter < 0.1

High lactose content Cream cheese 2–4 Cottage cheese 3.3

Lactose content in dairy products in g/100 g Low lactose content **Butter 0.6**

High lactose content Buttermilk 4
Ice cream 5–7
Yogurt 3–3.5
Kefir 3.5–6
Condensed milk 9.3 Cow milk 4.5–5.5 Milk powder 35–50 Quark 2–4
Cream 3–4
Sour cream 2–3
Goat milk 4.2

What Other Foods Contain Lactose?

Lactose is found in many industrially processed foods because lactose has a positive effect on the consistency of the food. It is a favorable filler and it becomes brownish in color when heated. This brownish color is one reason why lactose is added in the production of sausages. Particularly in the case of industrially processed foods, it is important to study the ingredients. Small quantities of lactose are also consumed with medicines since lactose is used as a carrier and filler in drug manufacturing. The lactose content of some drugs is indeed very high, but since tablets are absorbed only in small quantities little lactose is absorbed in this way.

What You Should Know About Yogurt?

Yogurt is high in lactose. However, if you do not want to do eliminate yogurt, you can look out for a few things that make some yogurts better tolerated than others. The FODMAP in yogurt is lactose, and its content can vary considerably in yogurt. The fluctuations depend on the manufacturing conditions. Lactose is degraded by the enzyme lactase in yogurt bacteria cultures. The longer these cultures can work, the lower the lactose content of the final product. Using your own yogurt machine, you can influence the time of production and let the yogurt cultures work 14 hours, or even as long as 18 hours, instead of 10 hours. This makes yogurt lower in lactose and therefore more digestible. When purchasing yogurt, make sure that it has not been pasteurized or heated, because this kills off all bacteria. Buy yogurt that contains living bacteria since they continue to split lactose in your intestines and thus exert a positive effect on digestion. If you choose to make your own yoghurt, you can use lactose-free milk. In this milk, the lactose is split into glucose and galactose. These two sugars do not cause digestive problems. Because of the glucose and galactose content, this yogurt tastes somewhat sweeter. It is important to note that for the production of yogurt made from lactose-free milk, a different yogurt culture is needed than for yogurt made from cow's milk. This yogurt culture is available at food health stores; alternatively, you can start your yogurt culture with cultures made from fresh, non-heat treated, lactose-free yogurt.

Is The Fodmap Share In Our Diet Increasing?

Yes, the share of FODMAPs in our diet is increasing for a variety of reasons. On the one hand, our dietary habits are changing towards more industrially processed foods and soft drinks. Both are sources of additional fructose. Fructose is used for sweetening here. But our consumption of fruits and fruit juices is also changing. Eating more fruit goes hand in hand with higher a consumption of FODMAPs, and FODMAPs in fruit juices are absorbed in very high concentrations. The changes in consumption are particularly evident in the case of various sugars. While the consumption of table sugar is declining and the consumption of lactose remains stable, the consumption of fructose is steadily increasing. Likewise, the increase in the consumption of polyols, i.e. sugar substitutes, in our diet can be explained by our altered nutritional behavior. The rising consumption of beverages, especially sweet drinks, and the rising consumption of low-calorie foodstuffs, are driving a higher consumption of sugar substitutes. This is especially evident in the case of beverages. 25 years ago, we did not know low-calorie or calorie-free drinks, meanwhile they have become standard. Another reason for the increase in FODMAPs in our diet is the trend towards industrially processed foods and fast food. These products are high in FODMAPs due to their high content of fructose and polyols.

! The share of FODMAPs in our diet is increasing due to:
- more industrially processed foods
- more soft drinks

- more low-calorie foods
- more snacks high in FODMAPs

Another trend in our diet leads to an increase in the daily FODMAP intake. A large part of the daily energy intake is nowadays provided by snacks, sweets or power bars. All these "intermediate meals" are high in FODMAPs. The type of foods we tend to consume on a daily basis has also changed. The share of pasta products, pizzas, cakes, cereals, pastries and products with a high fruit content has more than doubled over the last 20 years.
The amount of fructans consumed has also changed. Fructans are undoubtedly beneficial in food production. They improve the texture and stability of the food. Occasionally, food is marketed as a beneficial product due to its fructan content and hence fiber content. The fructan-potato is an example. In the end, however, all these fructan additions also change the daily consumed FODMAP quantity. While most cereal products contain a high share of fructans, the rice plant cannot synthesize fructans. Rice is therefore fructan-free. This is one reason why rice diets are very well tolerated by patients with digestive problems. Foods with added fructans can be identified, for example, by the label oligosaccharides, fructo-oligosaccharides or chicory.

What About Meat, Fish, Chicken, Fats And Oils?

Sources of protein such as meat, fish and chicken, as well as fats and oils, contain hardly any FODMAPs. This is because these foods contain hardly any carbohydrates. Therefore, these foods can be freely consumed by patients on a low-FODMAP diet. It should, however, be noted that the ingredients added during processing such as sauces, marinades or a dough coat do contain FODMAPs. Hence, their FODMAP content should be considered.

How To Assess The Ready-Made Products?

You will encounter difficulties in assessing the FODMAP content of the ready-to-use or ready-made products. Finished products which are offered in cans, dried or also frozen, but also sauces and dressings, contain a lot of FODMAPs and what is more, they often contain retrograded starch. Currently, the FODMAP content of these dishes is not indicated on the packaging.

! Fish, fats and oils, and meat are low in FODMAPs or FODMAP-free. Sauces, marinades and dough coat, however, may contain FODMAPs.

It is best to avoid such products if you are on a low-FODMAP diet, since this will allow you to have the best control over your diet. If you do not want to do without such dishes, you should carefully study the ingredients to assess the food. Please pay particular attention to ingredients such as fructose, sweeteners, onion and garlic, as these are often added in large amounts.

How Many Fodmaps Are In Hot Drinks?

Coffee contains only a low amount of FODMAPs and can be consumed as part of the diet. An exception is instant coffee, which is high in FODMAPs. It should be noted, however, that the added coffee cream or the added milk is high in FODMAPs and should be avoided. If you drink your coffee with milk, use lactose-free milk or a low-FODMAP substitute milk instead of cow's milk that is high in FODMAPs. Apart from the FODMAP content assessment, you should also remember that caffeine stimulates peristalsis and can therefore cause or intensify digestive problems. Therefore, the daily amount of coffee should be limited to a maximum of three cups, or even less if you suffer from digestive problems, regardless of the FODMAP content. No FODMAP assessment has yet been carried out for coffee substitute products; due to their chicory or malt content, these substitute products are, however, to be regarded as high in FODMAPs.

The evaluation of teas is not as easy as the evaluation of coffee because there are so many varieties. Peppermint tea, green tea, herbal tea and black tea are considered to be low in FODMAPs. Tea varieties high in FODMAPs are oolong tea, fennel tea and chamomile tea. In addition, the longer the tea bag sits in the cup, the higher the FODMAP content. This is important for chai tea and some herbal teas, so beware of leaving the tea bag in too long. Cocoa is low in FODMAPs and therefore suitable, if water, rice milk or lactose-free milk is used in the preparation of the hot beverage. When cow's milk is used, it must be taken into account that cow's milk is high in FODMAPs.

FODMAP content of teas

Low in FODMAPs
Chai tee (tea bag left in for a short time) Green tea Herbal tea (tea bag left in for a short time) Dandelion tea (tea bag left in for a short time) Peppermint tea Black tea (tea bag left in for a short time) White tea

Medium in FODMAPs
Chai tee (tea bag left in for a long time) Dandelion tea (tea bag left in for a long time) Black tea (tea bag left in for a long time)

High in FODMAPs
Fennel tea
Chamomile tea
Herbal tea (tea bag left in for a long time) Oolong tea

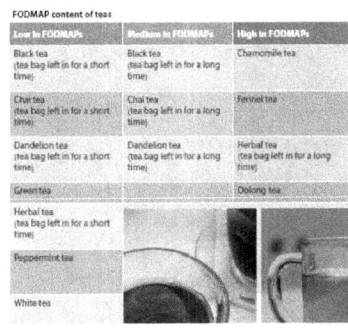

How Many Fodmaps Are In Chocolate?

Cocoa is low in FODMAPs and contributes little to the FODMAP content of chocolate. The FODMAPs in chocolate come from lactose. Therefore, dark and bitter chocolates, i.e. chocolates with a high cocoa content, are well-suited, while milk chocolate and white chocolate should best be avoided.

How Many Fodmaps Are Contained In Sweets And Soft Drinks?

Large amounts of sugar substitutes are hiding in sweets. Sugar substitutes of the polyol type are frequently used. Next time you buy a chewing gum or peppermint drops, review the package and you will find polyols listed. A chewing gum probably does not cause any digestive problems, but several of these sweets spread throughout the day contribute significantly to the FODMAP burden. The same applies to low-calorie soft drinks. Frequently, polyols are used as sugar substitutes in these drinks.

Does food preparation/processing change the FODMAP content?

The content of FODMAPs in a foodstuff changes with the preparation. Strong heating results in the decomposition of FODMAPs and thus a reduction in the FODMAP content. Factors such as the preparation temperature, the type (cooking, roasting, microwave) and the duration of the preparation all play a role. The extent to which the FODMAP content is changed by the different methods of preparation is unknown for most foodstuffs. Hence, the preparation is currently not yet addressed by the nutritional recommendations. This is likely to change in the future.

It is interesting that canned foods can release part of the FODMAPs, the so-called watersoluble FODMAPs, into the liquid used in the canning process. If vinegar is contained in the preserving liquid, this effect is further intensified by the acid contained therein. If, for example, canned onions are served, the liquid should be poured off in order to remove at least some of the FODMAPs.

However, the FODMAP content of certain foods can also increase during preparation, such as when drying fruits. Drying not only deprives the fruit of water, which results in an increase in FODMAPs per unit weight, but it can also result in additional FODMAP formation such as fructans formation, which are not contained in the fresh fruit. For this reason, you should exercise caution especially with dried fruits during the low-FODMAP diet, and be very careful when re-introducing food in phase 2.

! When fruits are dried, the share on FODMAPs per unit of weight increases. Often, additional FODMAPs, such as fructans, are generated by drying.

How Do I Replace Onions And Garlic?

It is not easy to eliminate onions and garlic from our diet. Onions and garlic are needed in many recipes as flavorers or flavor enhancers, and we have gotten used to the good taste. Unfortunately, onions and garlic are very high in FODMAPs and should best be avoided, or consumed in very small amounts when on the diet.
If you do not want to do without onions and garlic,

more precisely their fine taste, use a trick. FODMAPs are hardly soluble in oil. You can fry onions and garlic in oil and then remove them from the oil after a short time. The taste is partly transferred to the oil that can be used to prepare dishes, but the high-FODMAP onion and garlic themselves are not consumed. If this is too cumbersome, you can also buy oils that contain onion or garlic flavor. In the case of clear oils, only the taste, but not the onion and garlic, or their FODMAPs, is included. Another way to replace garlic and onion is to use the Ayurvedic spice (asafoetida) which, unlike onions and garlic, does not leave odors.

What Type Of Bread Is Low In Fodmaps?

The FODMAP content of bread depends mainly on the flour used. While bread made from wheat, barley or rye flour is considered to be high in FODMAPs and should be avoided, bread made from oatmeal or spelt flour using leaven is relatively low in FODMAPs. Bread dough that is prepared according to the traditional leavening method, i.e. using yeasts in combination with lactobacilli with a longer leavening time, is somewhat lower in FODMAPs since the yeasts and lactobacilli degrade a larger share of FODMAPs contained in the grain, thereby reducing the FODMAP content. Ask your baker for leavening times and select bread made of flour that is low in FODMAPs and prepared according to the traditional leavening method.

An elegant way to control the FODMAP content of bread is to prepare it yourself. In doing so, you can use grain low in FODMAPs or use alternatives low in FODMAPs such as corn flour, rice flour, or potato starch. In the above table there are numerous alternatives from which bread can be made. If you have nothing against square bread, you can simplify your low-FODMAP life with a bread baking machine. In 2-3 minutes, all the ingredients are mixed together, and the built-in time switches simplify your life and provide you with fresh bread for breakfast that will bolster your quality of life in addition to providing you with a FODMAP-free alternative. Since you do not need to eat entirely FODMAP-free, but merely low in FODMAPs, you need to replace only a part of the wheat flour with, for example, oatmeal. Such breads taste better than, for example, gluten-free breads.

FODMAP content of grain

Low in FODMAPs
Spelt flour (FODMAP content depends on the preparation) Oatmeal

High in FODMAPs Barley flour
Unripe spelt grain Rye flour
Wheat flour
Triticale flour

FODMAP content of grain alternatives

Low-FODMAP alternatives Arrowroot
Buckwheat
Millet
Potato starch/ potato flour Corn starch/ corn flour
Quinoa
Rice flour
Tapioca starch (from cassava)

Unsuitable alternatives Amaranth
Pea flour
Lupine flour

Dietary   fiber

Dietary fibers are an important part of the diet. They serve to regulate bowel function and bowel volume. The ability of the dietary fiber to bind water in the intestine plays a role in this process. Dietary fiber is a type of carbohydrate that your body cannot digest; it usually comes from plant sources.

Bulking   agents,   binders   and   stabilizers

Bulking agents, binders and stabilizers are added to foodstuffs to improve their texture. Most of these substances are not FODMAPs, so you do not need to limit them. This applies particularly to agar agar, carrageenan and gelatin. Pectin, xanthan gum and guar gum , as well as other stabilizers, cause bloating when consumed in large quantities. Hence, you should limit their consumption to a reasonable level.

Sweeteners

Sweetning is easy in the low-FODMAP diet. You should simply avoid all artificial sweeteners that are polyols. These sweeteners end with the letters -ol, and you will find their alternative names and their European E-number for food labeling listed in the following table. Other sweeteners such as the natural sweetener Stevia (E 960) and sweeteners not ending in -ol, e.g. aspartame (E 951), may be used.

If you do not use sweeteners but prefer natural sugars, you should use sucrose-based sugars (granulated sugar) or glucose-based sugars (glucose, dextrose). Maple sirup, cane sirup and sugar beet sirup are also suitable. Honey and corn sirup are not suitable for sweetening for they both contain a high fructose content.

FODMAP content of sweeteners Low in FODMAPs
Acesulfame-K, E 950
Aspartame, E 951
Aspartame-Acesulfame, E 962 Cyclamate, E 952
Neohesperidine-DC, E 959
Neotame, E 961
Saccharine, E 954
Stevia, E 960
Sucralose, E 955
Thaumatin, E 957

High in FODMAPs
Erythrite (Erythritol), E 968 Glycerol, E 422 Isomalt (Isomaltol), E 953 Lactit (Lactitol), E 966 Maltit (Maltitol), E 965 Mannit (Mannitol), E 421 Sorbit (Sorbitol), E 420 Xylit (Xylitol), E 967

Spices And Herbs

Spices and herbs are used only in small quantities in the preparation of meals and are therefore not restricted. Many of the spices have also not yet been investigated for their FODMAP content. Ready-to-serve seasonings and sauces should be avoided due to the large number of ingredients that are sometimes poorly identifiable. It is also best to avoid stock cubes, clear soup powders and seasoning sauces such as soy sauce, particularly larger quantities thereof, while smaller amounts are OK. By contrast, you are fee to use anise, basil, cayenne pepper, curry, dill, ginger, cardamom, chervil, coriander, cumin, liquorice, lavender, marjoram, mint, nutmeg, cloves, oregano, peppers, parsley, pepper, thyme, chives, mustard, vanilla, juniper, cinnamon and lemongrass. You can season various dishes with fresh or dried spices and make them even more delicious.

! No Fodmap-Free Life, Please! The Handling Of Ready-To-Serve Products, Pastries And Drinks

There is no such thing as a FODMAP-free life, and it is not necessary either. The diet should be low in FODMAPs, but not FODMAP-free, which is also not possible. Phase 1 of the diet is strictly low in FODMAPs, while phase 2 is gradually more liberal in terms of restrictions, which means that you will try to reintroduce individual foods high in FODMAPs into your diet.

This is the moment when the question arises as to how to deal with our normal Western diet. The individual foods listed in the tables are very easy to avoid or consume. It is more difficult to permanently avoid industrially processed mixed food. Very few of us really want that. A few simple tips will help you incorporate industrially processed foods, pastries and drinks into your low-FODMAP life.

Sauces And Dressings

Sauces and dressings can be found in every refrigerator. It is hard to imagine a barbecue steak without barbecue sauce. You do not have to do without it! Just be sure to take much less dressing, the stress being on "much less". The steak does not have to float in sauce for you to enjoy the taste of it, and a fresh salad with just a touch of dressing simply tastes better.

Take note of the ingredients and avoid FODMAPs that you recognize. Since the exact quantities are usually not declared, you will have to try several products until you find the one that is most acceptable to you, including in terms of quantity. Health food stores regularly offer numerous sauces, dressings and seasonings that are lactose-free and gluten-free. These are suitable for a low-FODMAP diet because at least some of the FODMAPs are removed.

Baking And Baked Goods

Baking is certainly one of the biggest challenges because it is extremely difficult to find low-FODMAP cereal flour replacement products. This applies to baking cakes and bread, as well as all other foodstuffs where flour is used. There are many substitute flours, and you have learned about them at the beginning of this book. But not a single one of these substitute flours can really replace cereal flour and the gluten contained in it. Therefore, different strategies are needed to deal with this situation. One strategy is to avoid such baked goods as much as possible, and later on in phase 2 of the diet find out how much of these baking/flour products you can tolerate.

Ready-Made Gluten-Free Flour Mixtures

Another strategy is to find substitute flours such as gluten-free flours. This strategy is especially suitable for those who simply adore pastries and flour products. However, always check which flours and which additives are used, as there are also gluten-free substitute flours classified as high in FODMAPs. Some shops offer gluten-free flours at a cheaper price, especially if they are bought in larger quantities. These ready-made substitute flours can be used for baking just like wheat flour. The ready-made substitute flour usually consists of corn flour and rice flour, potato starch, corn starch and an adhesive (guar gum, carob kernel flour or xanthan gum). The ready-made substitute flour is slightly more expensive than wheat flour, but cheaper than the next strategy, which is making your own substitute flour. To mix your substitute flour yourself. You will need a mixture of at least three different flours.

Flour Mixtures For Bread

For breads or firmer baked products, a possible mixture consists of two parts of rice flour, one part of corn starch, one part of corn flour or soy flour, and two coated teaspoons of substitute gluten per 500 grams of flour. Xanthan, guar gum or carob gum may be used as a substitute gluten. 2 tsp xanthan correspond to approx. 3 tsp guar gum or 3 tsp carob gum. Xanthan gives a rubbery texture, which is not for everyone, while guar gum and carob gum impart a less solid texture. Depending on the firmness, the amounts of these gluten substitutes are to be increased or decreased to suit your taste. Corn starch can be found in every supermarket because the starch we usually buy at the supermarket is corn starch. Corn starch can alternatively be replaced by potato starch. Potato starch is called potato flour in many supermarkets.

Flour mixtures low in FODMAPs

For breads and pastries
500 g of rice flour
250 g of soy flour *
125 g of potato starch
125 g of corn starch
2 tsp of xanthan gum

For breads and pastries
450 g of rice flour
50 g of grated hazelnuts
250 g of corn starch
175 g of soy flour *
100 g of tapioca flour 3 tsp of guar gum

For cakes and pastries with egg
450 g of rice flour
50 g of grated hazelnuts
250 g of corn starch
250 g of potato starch
3 tsp of carob gum

* Soy flour contains oligosaccharides. In small quantities, however, most patients with irritable bowel syndrome tolerate it well. Test your individual tolerance threshold.

Flour mixture for cakes and pastries with egg
For cakes with baked eggs, a flour mixture of one part of soy flour, one part of corn starch and two parts of rice flour can also be used. The more different flours you mix, the more similar the characteristics of your flour will resemble those of wheat flour. For example, there are three possible flours listed in this book. However, those who find this mixing too cumbersome can obtain gluten-free flours. For pastries such as Christmas cookies, it is often helpful to increase the share of rice flour a bit. Tastes are different, so you are free to experiment a bit with flour. You will find that baked goods from substitute flour dry out more quickly. If you want your products to be slightly moister, you can replace a portion of the rice flour with ground hazelnuts.

Drinks

There are non-alcoholic and alcoholic drinks. Drinking only water, ideally mildly carbonated or non-carbonated, would be most compatible with a low-FODMAP diet. Carbonated water is not suitable for

your bowels.
Fruit and vegetable juices are high in FODMAPs since they are concentrated. If you drink fruit and vegetable juice, be sure to choose low-FODMAP variants, limit the amount to half a glass and dilute the juice with water, then you'll derive more benefit. In moderation, you do not have to do without orange juice.
If you like to drink milk, it will be hard on you. Try to keep consumption to a minimum or to change to alternatives such as lactose-free milk or rice milk. Admittedly, however, they do not taste the same.
Lemonades, and especially lemonades high in fructose or substitute sugars, are unsuitable. More information can be found in the earlier "Fructose" section of this Guide, as well as in the section "How many FODMAPs are contained in sweets and soft drinks?".
The assessment of warm and hot drinks can be found in the section "How many FODMAPs are in hot beverages?" of this Guide.
As for alcoholic beverages, alcohol should generally be consumed only in moderation or not at all. If you want an alcoholic drink, then beer is rather unsuitable because of the grain and malt content. It should be drunk in small quantities, i.e. a small glass at the most. Wine and sparkling wines are high in FODMAPs, with the FODMAP content rising with the sweetness level. So if you absolutely must have a glass of wine, then

select one that is as dry as possible. Other spirits are harmless, but such high-percentage spirits are also not consumed in large quantities. Exercise caution when drinking mixed alcoholic drinks, paying particular attention to the other ingredients.

Is The Low-Fodmap Diet Compatible With Other Diets??

The low-FODMAP diet is generally compatible with most other diets because you have a wide range of foods to choose from. The situation may become intricate, however, if you have to consume foods high in FODMAPs due to another illness. An example is diabetes because it often requires sugar substitutes that are high in FODMAPs. Another example are liver diseases where special diets are to be observed. If you have to follow a special diet for medical reasons, you should consult a nutritionist before starting the lowFODMAP as part of your individual diet plan.

Fodmaps And The Vegetarian Or Vegan Diet

This also applies, with certain limitations, to people who are strictly vegan or vegetarian. A vegan or vegetarian diet is only partially compatible with a low-FODMAP diet, because dairy products and legumes that are high in FODMAPs are frequently consumed in order to meet the protein requirements of vegetarians. Vegetarians and vegans have to plan their diets very carefully. In order to avoid deficiencies, they may have to adopt a less strict low-FODMAP diet. Nutritional counseling is recommended in order to avoid deficiencies.

Part 2

Vegetarian And Vegan

Vegetarian and Vegan

P.113 - Halloumi Kebabs with Asian Dressing

P.114 - Vegetable Tartlets

P.115 - Three Cheese Broccoli Bake

P.116 - Halloumi Burgers

P.117 - Aubergine Parmigiana

P.118 - Vegetable Bake with a Cheddar and Pumpkin Seed Crust

P.119 - Ramen with Crispy Tofu

P.120 - Vegetable Pasta Bake

P.121 - Griddled Courgette Salad

P.122 - Macaroni 'Cheese'

P.123 - Whipped Feta Dip with Vegetable Crudités

Halloumi Kebabs With Asian Dressing (Serves 2)

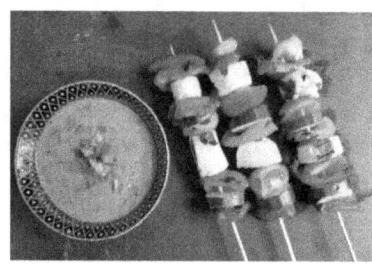

Halloumi seems to divide people into two camps. There are those who love its firm, chewy, creamy texture and others who think its 'squeaky' texture is an abomination within the fromage world. I fall into the former congregation. Although halloumi contains lactose, it is low FODMAP at a serving of 50g, although you can increase this portion to 100g if you're okay with digesting lactose.

Halloumi goes well with most vegetables, particularly if you chargrill them, because it provides the perfect slightly bitter contrast to the soft creaminess of the halloumi cheese. I pair my halloumi kebabs with an Asian dressing that's really easy to knock up. The dressing really complements the halloumi kebabs and allows the individual flavours of the kebab vegetables to come through without being overpowered.

Ingredients for the halloumi kebabs:

100g halloumi (cut into thick cubes)
120g courgette (cut into discs)
100g red bell pepper (cut into bite-sized pieces)
100g green bell pepper (cut into bite-sized pieces)
1 common tomato

Ingredients for the Asian dressing:

1/2 a red chilli (but add more or less to suit your own taste)
2 tbsps soy sauce (or tamari – a gluten-free version)
2 tsps brown sugar
2 tbsps lime juice
1 tbsp sesame oil
2 tbsps fresh coriander (finely chopped)
2 tbsps peanut butter

Method:

Prepare your kebab ingredients as directed and divide them onto six kebab skewers.

(If you're cooking these kebabs in the house, preheat a griddle pan until hot and cook them on all sides until charred. If you're cooking them on the BBQ place them over medium-hot coals and rotate them periodically until they're cooked all the way round.)

Make your Asian dressing by mixing all of the dressing ingredients together in a bowl until blended.

Once your kebabs are cooked serve them with the dressing on the side.

Vegetable Tartlets (Serves 4)

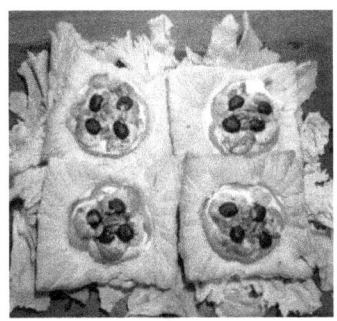

Ingredients:
300g ready-rolled gluten-free puff pastry
100g sweet potato (cut into 4 thin discs)
6 cherry tomatoes (halved)
50g green bell pepper (sliced into rounds)
1 beaten egg
30g grated parmesan
8 black olives (sliced)
100g feta (cubed)
1 tbsp rice milk
1 carrot (cut into thin strips or grated)
10g of green spring onion tips (chopped)
1/2 tsp ground black pepper
1/2 tsp dried oregano
2 tbsps pumpkin seeds

These vegetable tartlets are essentially just small quiches, but they're lighter than a normal quiche thanks to the use of puff pastry instead of shortcrust and the omission of any meat.

You could make these in individual tartlet tins if you like, but I just make mine in a Yorkshire pudding tin and it works just fine.

I serve these vegetable tartlets with some homemade potato wedges and a fresh green salad and it makes for a very substantial meal.

The tartlets are a great combination of crispy puff pastry that encases a selection of soft, fresh vegetables and creamy feta and parmesan cheese.

They're an excellent option for a meat-free meal.

Method:

Prepare the vegetables as directed and preheat your oven to 220C/200C Fan/Gas Mark 7.

Unroll your puff-pastry sheet and cut it into four quarters. Place the puff pastry in your tins and trim if needed. (I don't bother, life's too short.)

Whisk the egg with the rice milk, black pepper, oregano and parmesan.

Cook your discs of sweet potato in the microwave until soft and then put one in the bottom of each tartlet and put the feta cheese, tomato halves, slices of green pepper, carrot and chopped spring onion on top.

Pour the egg mixture into the tartlets and top with the sliced olives and pumpkin seeds.

Bake in the oven for 20-25 mins until the pastry is puffed up and golden brown. Serve.

Three Cheese Broccoli Bake (Serves 4-6)

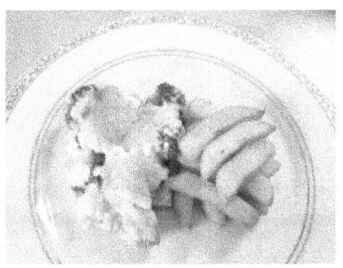

To make this three cheese broccoli bake I use my recipe for dairy-free cheese sauce which is based on nutritional yeast (aka 'nooch') and if you choose to use non-dairy versions of the cheeses you can easily make a completely dairy-free version. If you'd like to try reintroducing broccoli into your diet then I'd highly recommend this three cheese broccoli bake. It's rich, creamy and extremely cheesy, but remains quite light thanks to the fresh broccoli. You can serve it on its own as a main meal or as a side dish, but we have it with chips on the side and salad and it's a great mid-week meal.

Ingredients:
300g whole broccoli
40g grated lactose-free cheddar cheese (or non-dairy version)
180g cubed feta cheese (or non-dairy version)
30g grated parmesan (or non-dairy version)
Black pepper

Ingredients for the non-dairy cheese sauce:

1 tbsp non-dairy butter
1 tbsp gluten-free flour
200ml rice milk
60g (4 tbsps) nutritional yeast (nooch)
1 tsp cornflour dissolved in 2 tbsps water
Salt and pepper (to taste)

Method:

Preheat your oven to 200C/180C Fan/400F/Gas Mark 6.

Cook the broccoli and then place it in a casserole dish.

To make the sauce, put the butter and flour in a saucepan over a medium heat and make a roux by stirring it until it has melted down.

Whisk in a little of the rice milk at a time until a smooth sauce is formed.

Add the nutritional yeast and cornflour mixture and stir in. Cook until the sauce is thickened. Taste and season with black pepper.

Pour the sauce over the broccoli and add the feta, if you're using it. Scatter the cheddar on top and then the parmesan.

Bake it in the oven for 25-30 mins until it is golden brown and the cheese is crispy on top then serve.

Halloumi Burgers (Serves 4)

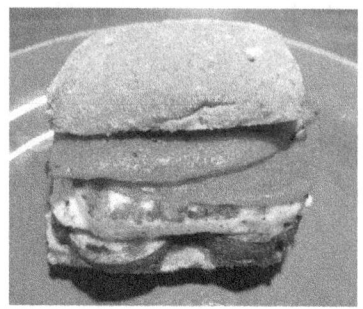

Ingredients:

160g halloumi (cut into 4 slices)
Red bell peppers in brine
4 gluten-free burger rolls
100g courgette (cut into discs)

If you're a vegetarian, halloumi is one of the tastiest cheeses around to use for a veggie burger alternative if you're having a barbecue.

I like to serve thick slices of halloumi that have been griddled on top of warmed gluten-free buns along with griddled fresh courgettes and strips of red bell peppers.

Other toppings can include chargrilled oyster mushrooms (low FODMAP in portions of up to 75g) and jalapeños.

Method:

Heat a griddle pan and griddle your courgette slices on both sides until they are soft and keep to one side.

Griddle the halloumi slices on both sides until they are hot.

Cut your roll in half and spread it with mayo and layer the courgette on the base, followed by a slice of halloumi and top it with a slice of red pepper.

Serve.

Aubergine Parmigiana (Serves 4)

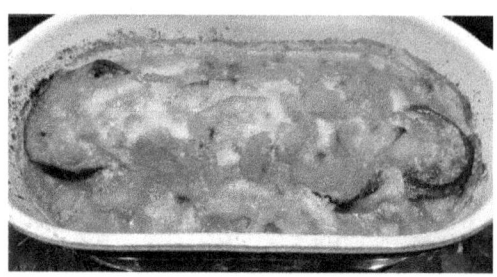

I'll be the first to admit that this photo doesn't really do aubergine parmigiana justice, but although it's a difficult meal to photograph it really is divine. Aubergine parmigiana consists of slices of tender aubergine which are layered with grated parmesan and chopped tomatoes and then topped with seasoned herby breadcrumbs. It's brilliant as a main meal or as a side.

For the aubergine parmigiana:

300g aubergine (sliced)
1/2 tsp asafoetida
1 tsp dried oregano
360g tinned chopped tomatoes
100g grated parmesan
160g mozzarella (sliced)

1/2 tsp salt
1/2 tsp pepper
2 tsps red wine vinegar

For the topping:

100g gluten-free breadcrumbs (roughly 2 slices worth)
1 tbsp of olive oil
20g grated parmesan
1 tsp dried oregano

Method:

Preheat your oven to 200C/180C Fan/400F/Gas Mark 6.

Slice the aubergine into 1 cm thick discs and use a hot griddle pan to fry the aubergine until it is slightly soft then leave it to one side.

To make the sauce: Put the tinned tomatoes, asafoetida, oregano, salt, pepper and red wine vinegar in a saucepan and heat through.

Get your casserole dish and put a small amount of sauce on the base, followed by some of the grated parmesan cheese (reserve 2 tbsps of parmesan for the topping) and then a layer of aubergine.

Repeat until all of the ingredients have been used and put the mozzarella on top.

Mix the breadcrumbs with the 2 tbsps of parmesan and tbsp of olive oil and sprinkle on top before baking in the oven for half an hour until the top is golden and crispy.

Vegetable Bake With A Cheddar And Pumpkin Crust (Serves 6)

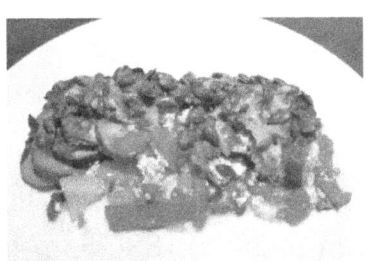

This vegetable bake with a cheddar and pumpkin crust makes a cracking vegetarian dinner because it is fresh and light while remaining filling and substantial. It's formed from sliced discs of courgette and aubergine that surround sliced bell peppers and is topped with a rich tomato sauce. The crisp baked cheddar and pumpkin crust enhances the dish by providing a crunchy texture contrast with the soft, tender vegetables. We have this for dinner almost weekly!

Ingredients:
300g courgettes (sliced into thin discs)
1 red bell pepper
1 small aubergine – around 200g (sliced into thin discs)
2 common tomatoes

400g tinned chopped tomatoes
1 tsp dried oregano
1 tbsp dried chives
2 tsps red wine vinegar
400g feta (thinly sliced)
100g grated mature cheddar cheese
50g pumpkin seeds

Method:

Preheat your oven to 200C/180C Fan/400F/Gas Mark 6 and have a large casserole dish to hand.

Prepare your vegetables as directed and then place slices of vegetables in the casserole dish interspersing them with slices of feta cheese.

Pour the chopped tomatoes into a jug and stir in the dried chives, oregano and red wine vinegar before pouring it over the vegetables and feta.

Scatter the top of the vegetable bake with the grated cheddar and then the pumpkin seeds before baking it in the oven for 40-50 mins.

Ramen With Crispy Tofu (Serves 4)

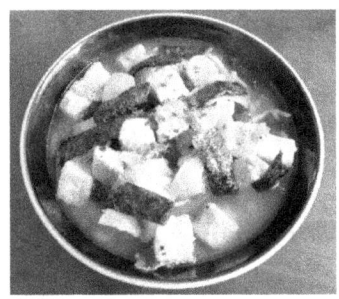

Ingredients:
1 carrot (cut into thin ribbons)
1 red bell pepper (sliced thinly)
2 pints of low FODMAP vegetable stock
2 tsps soy sauce (or gluten-free tamari)
4 tsps fish sauce
1 tbsp fresh ginger (minced)
1 sheet of nori seaweed (cut into strips)
400g firm tofu (drained well and cubed)
2 tbsps cornflour
Salt and pepper
1 tbsp sesame oil
Enough gluten-free noodles for 4 people
Pickled ginger

Although I'm not the hugest fan of tofu I really like this ramen with crispy tofu because the tofu is well-seasoned and has a delicious crunchy coating which contrasts beautifully with the tender tofu inside.

I like to build my ramen bowl around a base of gluten-free noodles which are topped with lots of sliced red pepper and pickled ginger.

You could also add other vegetables, such as whole broccoli florets, which are low FODMAP in servings of up to 70g per person.

Method:

Place the cornflour on a plate and season it with salt and pepper.

Toss the tofu cubes in the flour until they are coated.

Put a large saucepan over a medium heat and add the vegetable stock, carrots, peppers, soy sauce, fish sauce and ginger and bring to a gentle simmer.

Add the noodles to the vegetable stock and let them cook.

While the noodles are cooking, heat the sesame oil in a frying pan and when it's hot fry the tofu cubes until they are golden brown.

Serve the ramen in bowls with the crispy tofu on top and strips of nori and pickled ginger.

Vegetable Pasta Bake (Serves 4-6)

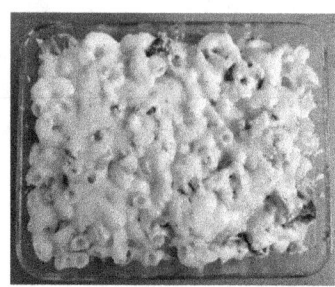

Ingredients:

2 tbsps. oil
1 red bell pepper (deseeded and sliced)
1 yellow bell pepper (deseeded and sliced)
10 black olives (halved)
30g sundried tomatoes (finely chopped)
320g tinned chopped tomatoes
50g whole broccoli (cut into small pieces)
50g green beans (cut into small pieces)
50g oyster mushrooms (cut into small pieces)
1 tsp Worcestershire sauce
150g grated cheddar cheese (or non-dairy version)
Jalapeños (optional)

Sometimes if I've got a lot of little portions of vegetables left over in my fridge that need to be used up I like to throw them into a pasta oven bake. When they're mixed into tender pasta shapes and a rich tangy fresh tomato sauce and then topped with a scattering of grated cheddar cheese they are transformed from fridge leftovers into a very substantial and highly delicious evening meal.

I tend to like this flavour combination of broccoli, green beans and oyster mushrooms, but you can add other low FODMAP veggies as you like, but be careful not to over stack your FODMAP quota by using too many vegetables from the same FODMAP group.

This vegetable pasta bake can be eaten as a very filling meal on its own, but I like to serve it with a stack of crispy chips because they add a lovely crunch to the meal.

Method:

Cook the broccoli in a bowl with a little bit of water in it and pierced cling film on top in the microwave until it is tender. Drain.

Put a large frying pan over a medium heat and add the oil and then fry the peppers, green beans, mushrooms, olives and sundried tomatoes until soft.

Add the broccoli, chopped tomatoes and Worcestershire sauce. Simmer while you make the pasta.

Drain the pasta once it's cooked to your liking and pour it into a large casserole dish.

Add the vegetable ragù from the frying pan, stir it through the pasta and top with the grated cheese.

Bake it in the oven until the cheese is golden brown and then serve.

Griddled Courgette Salad (Serves 4)

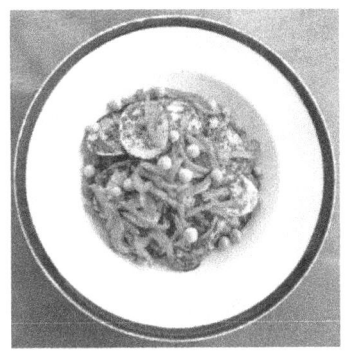

Ingredients:
240g courgettes (maximum prepared weight)
2 tbsps. olive oil
The zest and juice of 1 lemon
30g peas
1 red bell pepper (deseeded and thinly sliced)
Dried chilli flakes (optional)
Salt and pepper

I have to be honest, this salad began its life as a side dish to accompany a lasagne one evening, but it was so tasty that I couldn't let it not become a star in its own right.

As it was summer when I first made this salad I used fresh garden peas, but you can just use frozen peas which have been boiled and then cooled in a bit of cold water.

This salad is bright and fresh and enlivens any mealtime!

Method:

Put a griddle pan over a medium-high heat.

Cut the ends off the courgettes and cut them into 1cm thick discs before dusting both sides of them with salt and pepper and brushing them with olive oil.

Once the griddle is hot fry the red pepper in a little bit of oil until soft and then remove it and keep to one side.

Put the courgettes in the griddle and scatter half of the lemon zest on top along with half of the juice.

Leave them to cook until dark stripes have formed on the bottom before flipping them over and repeating. (If you think they're getting too dark before cooking though then turn the heat down.)

Once the courgettes are tender remove them and put them in a bowl along with the red pepper strips. Scatter with the peas and chilli (if you're using them) and season to taste before serving.

Macaroni 'Cheese' (Serves 4)

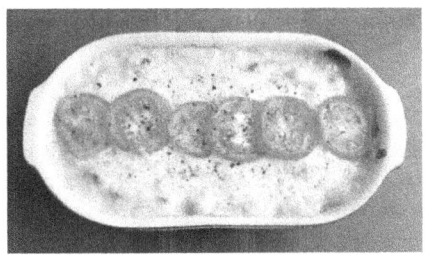

I first discovered nutritional yeast (also known as 'nooch') when I began eating dairy-free as a result of being diagnosed with a cow's milk protein allergy. Although I was really sceptical about its alleged cheese-like taste qualities it wasn't until I made my first nooch 'cheese' sauce that I was truly convinced. The nutritional yeast does have a mild cheesy flavour, but it also has a beautiful background nutty taste too, which makes it a winner in my book.

If you're not vegan or dairy-free you can just use lactose-free milk and grated cheddar in your cheese sauce instead of the nooch. Another ingredient which makes a lovely addition to the sauce is a teaspoon of Dijon mustard. Also, it's worth noting that you don't necessarily have to bake the dish because it can be served as cheese sauce coated pasta if you like.

Ingredients:
200g gluten-free macaroni
80g non-dairy cheddar 'cheese'
1 or 2 common tomatoes (sliced)

For the 'cheese' sauce:

600ml rice milk
50g non-dairy butter
50g gluten-free flour
4 tbsps. nutritional yeast flakes
Salt and pepper (to taste)
100g non-dairy cheddar 'cheese'

Method:

Start by boiling your pasta in salted water.

In the meantime, make a roux by placing a saucepan over a medium heat and melting the butter and flour together.

Stir them together for a minute or two and then slowly add the rice milk a little at a time, stirring all the while, until a smooth sauce is formed.

Continue to stir the sauce and add 80g of the non-dairy cheese and allow it to combine into the sauce. Season to taste.

Preheat your oven to 200C/180C Fan/400F/Gas Mark 6 and have a casserole dish at hand.

Once the pasta is done to your liking, drain it and put it in a casserole dish before mixing the cheese sauce into the pasta.

Scatter the rest of the grated cheese on top and top with sliced common tomatoes.

Bake in the oven until the cheese is golden brown and then serve.

Whipped Feta Dip With Vegetable Crudités
(Serves 4)

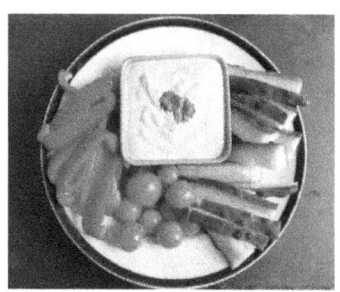

This is an excellent dip to serve on the side of a main meal or to have as a light lunch and although I have named it as a feta dip I've made a vegan version of this countless times with non-dairy soft cheese and it's just as tasty.

I like to serve it with low FODMAP vegetable sticks on the side, such as slices of bell pepper, cucumber, carrot and cherry tomatoes. (Cherry tomatoes are low FODMAP in servings of no more than 75g per person).

This dip is a firm favourite with kids and adults alike, so all you've got to stress is that there's no double-dipping!

Ingredients:
160g feta cheese
100ml lactose-free milk (or non-dairy version)
2 tbsps. chopped chives
2 tbsps. fresh oregano leaves
¼ tsp ground black pepper
1 tbsp. lemon juice

Method:

Simply mix all of the ingredients together until it forms a smooth dip consistency. Serve with low FODMAP vegetables.

Baking

Baking

P.126 - Rhubarb Cake with Lemon Sauce

P.127 - Strawberry Cake

P.128 - Gluten-Free Scones

P.129 - Lemon and Poppy Seed Pound Cake

P.130 - Palmiers

P.131 - Whoopie Pies

P.132 - Chocolate Orange Biscuits

P.133 - Dark Chocolate and Ginger Oaties

P.134 - Macadamia Nut Blondies

P.135 - Viennese Whirls

P.136 - Red Velvet Muffins

P.137 - Strawberry Turnovers

P.138 - Coffee and Walnut Cake

P.139 - Oat Crumblies

Rhubarb Cake With Lemon Sauce (Serves 8-10)

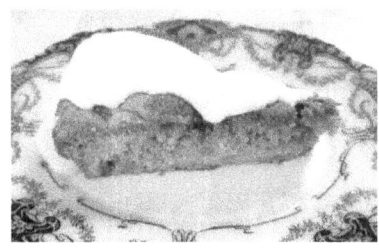

I baked this rhubarb cake with lemon sauce after I'd been given a couple of handfuls of fresh rhubarb stalks from my Dad. I had intended on making a rhubarb tatin (much like the quintessential apple tart tatin), but I couldn't be bothered waiting for my gluten-free puff pastry to defrost, so I just made it into a cake instead. I'll get around to the rhubarb tatin some time...

This rhubarb cake is incredibly moreish thanks to it being based around a soft, lemon-scented sponge that's loaded with fruity little chunks of soft, but tart, melting rhubarb and it goes wonderfully with the creamy and smooth lemon sauce that's made from a simple blend of lemon curd, icing sugar and cream cheese.

Ingredients for the Rhubarb Cake:

200g butter (or non-dairy version)
200g brown sugar
The zest of 1 lemon (or 1 tsp lemon extract)
3 eggs
150g gluten-free self-raising
1 tbsp dried ground ginger
1 tsp baking powder
1 tsp xanthan gum
400g rhubarb (washed and chopped into 1 cm chunks)

Ingredients for the Lemon Sauce:

150g lactose-free cream cheese
150g lemon curd
3 tbsps icing sugar

Method:

Preheat your oven to 180°C/170°C Fan/350°F/Gas Mark 4 and line a 20cm cake tin with greaseproof paper.

Measure the butter, sugar and lemon zest into a large mixing bowl and cream together. Add the eggs and whisk again. Add the flour, baking powder, dried ginger and xanthan gum and mix well.

Fold half of the rhubarb into the batter and pour it into the cake tin then scatter the rest of the rhubarb on top and bake it for 45-50 mins or until a skewer pushed into the middle of the cake comes out clean.

Leave it to cool and make the lemon sauce by placing the cream cheese, lemon curd and icing sugar in a jug or bowl and whisking together until a smooth sauce is formed. Once the cake has cooled serve it with the lemon sauce.

Strawberry Cake (Serves 6-8)

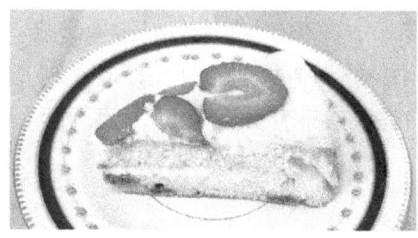

This strawberry cake is a gorgeously light little sponge which is peppered throughout with chunks of sweet strawberry and is sandwiched and topped with fluffy buttercream icing that's decorated with sliced fresh strawberries. All in all, it's an absolute celebration of the delicate fruit which is the strawberry.

Ingredients:
100g butter (or non-dairy version)
100g sugar
2 eggs
1 tsp vanilla extract
80g self-raising gluten-free flour
1/2 tsp baking powder
1/2 tsp xanthan gum
80g strawberries (chopped into quarters) and a couple to decorate the cake

For the buttercream icing:

100g butter (or non-dairy version)
150g icing sugar
2 tbsps non-dairy milk (or lactose-free milk)

Method:

Preheat your oven to 180C/160 Fan/350F/Gas Mark 5 and line a 9 inch cake tin with greaseproof paper.

Put your butter and sugar in a mixing bowl and whisk. Add the eggs and vanilla and whisk again until combined.

Add the flour, baking powder and xanthan gum and whisk until combined.

Gently fold the strawberries into the mixture (keep a couple aside to decorate the cake) and pour the batter into your tin.

Bake for 25-30 mins or until a skewer pushed into the middle of the cake comes out clean.

Leave to cool and make the buttercream icing by mixing all of the icing ingredients together until combined.

Once the cake is cool cut it in half horizontally. Place half of the icing on the bottom of the cake and then put the other half on top and top it with the rest of the icing.

Thinly slice the remaining strawberries and decorate the cake with them before serving.

Gluten-Free Scones (Makes 12)

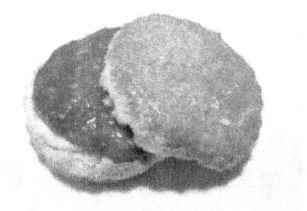

Ingredients:
250g self-raising gluten-free flour
1 tsp baking powder
1 tsp xanthan gum
50g sugar
90g butter (or non-dairy version)
100ml rice milk
1 small beaten egg (Optional)

Although this recipe for gluten-free scones makes just a standard sweet tea scone it can be adapted in many ways.

For instance, you can leave the sugar out and make herb and cheese scones to be eaten on their own with butter or to accompany a bowl of soup by adding

100g of cheddar cheese (or a non-dairy version) and 1 tsp of dried mixed herbs.

Another option is to add dried fruit to them, such as 50g of dried cranberries or even 100g of fresh blueberries or raspberries.

I brush the tops of my scones with a little beaten egg to give their tops a shine and a nice golden brown colour, but that's an optional step.

Method:

Preheat your oven to 220C/200C Fan/425F/Gas Mark 6 and have a greaseproof-papered baking tray to hand.

Measure all of the dry ingredients into a large mixing bowl and mix together.

Add the butter and rub it into the flour mixture until it resembles wet sand or fine breadcrumbs.

Add the milk and gently combine into a dough.

Roll out the dough on a floured surface and use a pastry cutter to cut out as many scones as you can get out of the dough, re-rolling as required. (If you don't have a pastry cutter you can just use a knife to cut the dough into squares or triangles. Thankfully, scones can be any shape you like!)

Once all of your scones are cut, brush the tops of them with a little beaten egg and then put them on the baking tray and bake them in the oven for 12-15 mins or until they are puffed up and golden brown.

Leave them to cool slightly before serving them warm with butter and low FODMAP jam.

Lemon And Poppy Seed Pound Cake (Makes 12 Slices)

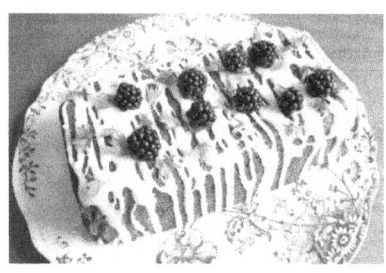

Pound cakes are so called because they are an American type of cake that uses a pound each of butter, sugar, flour and eggs to create the cake. They are normally baked in a loaf tin and drizzled with icing sugar or a sugar glaze and then served in slices. This lemon and poppy seed pound cake has a base of gluten-free flour and ground almonds, but although almonds become high FODMAP at servings of over 12g, this cake yields a total of 12 slices which keeps the FODMAP quota low.

Ingredients:
140g ground almonds
1 tbsp poppy seeds
100g gluten-free flour

2 tsps baking powder
1/2 tsp bicarbonate of soda
1 tsp xanthan gum
150g sugar
120ml vegetable oil
2 eggs
2 tsps lemon extract
120ml rice milk
2 tsps lemon juice

For decoration:

Icing sugar
Dried cornflowers

Method:

Preheat your oven to 180C/160 Fan/350F/Gas Mark 4 and line a two pound loaf tin with greaseproof paper.

In a large mixing bowl, mix all of your wet ingredients together and then mix in the dry ingredients.

Once it's all combined, pour your batter into the loaf tin, smooth it out and bake it in the oven for around 50 mins to an hour. Don't worry if it needs a little longer. (You'll know it's baked when a skewer pushed into the middle comes out clean.)

Once it's baked, let it cool on a cooling rack.

Make some icing by mixing icing sugar with a little water at a time until it just coats the back of a spoon. Once your cake is cool, drizzle it with some icing sugar and add any decoration you like. Serve.

Palmiers (Makes 8)

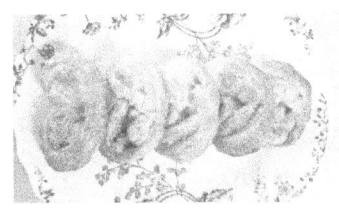

Ingredients:
1 block of gluten-free puff pastry (mine weighed 320g)
80g caster sugar (plus a little extra)
1 tsp ground cinnamon

If you don't already know, palmiers are French pastries that are made from sheets of puff pastry which are coated in sugar and cinnamon before being folded (or rolled) from each side into the middle to create the distinctive shape of a palmier.

Palmiers have to be one of the easiest biscuits you can make, mainly because if you buy a batch of puff pastry then most of the work is done for you.

It's literally just a case of rolling out the pastry, scattering it with a little water, sugar and cinnamon and then rolling it up before cutting it into slices. You can't get any easier than that!

If you make these palmiers you'll be rewarded with a batch of flaky, butter-enriched pastries which crumble and fracture into sweet shards of butteriness in your mouth while infusing it with a delicious blend of crisp, caramelised sugar and warm cinnamon flavours. These go fast in my house. I wonder how long they'll last in yours.

Method:

Preheat your oven to 200C/180C Fan/400F/Gas Mark 6 and line two baking trays with greaseproof paper.

Mix the cinnamon into the sugar and then roll out your puff pastry until it's a large rectangle and lightly wet it with a little cold water.

Scatter half of the sugar over the pastry and spread it until it's even then turn the pastry over, wet it again, and scatter the other half of the sugar over it and spread it until it's even.

Take the left and right sides of the pastry and fold them into the centre of the pastry so the two sides meet in the middle. Repeat once again and then fold the two sides together so that a large sausage shape is formed.

Turn the pastry horizontally and cut it into 1 cm thick slices before lying them on the baking trays with a generous gap between each palmier.

Scatter them with a little more caster sugar and then bake them in the oven for 12-15 mins or until puffed up and golden brown.

Leave on a cooling rack to cool slightly before eating.

Whoopie Pies (Makes 10)

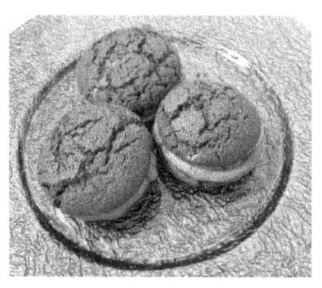

Ingredients:
220g dark brown sugar
120g fine polenta
50g gluten-free flour
90g ground almonds
50g cocoa powder
A pinch of salt
2 tsps baking powder
1/2 tsp of bicarbonate of soda
120g butter (or dairy-free version)
100g coconut oil (melted)
4 eggs
60ml rice milk

For the buttercream:

150g butter (or dairy-free version)
170g icing sugar
30g cocoa
1 tbsp rice milk

I've always loved whoopie pies, but sometimes shop-bought whoopie pies can be a bit too sickly because they have too much filling inside them and the quality of the buttercream icing often leaves a lot to be desired. The beauty of baking your own therefore, is that you can control the buttercream icing to baked sponge ratio to suit your own taste.

I make my whoopie pies traditional chocolate ones, but you can omit the cocoa powder and make them with other flavours instead, such as vanilla (using 1 tsp vanilla extract), lemon (using the zest of 1 lemon) or bake them as a plain sponge but sandwich them with strawberry jam as well as buttercream icing. One whoopie pie is a low FODMAP portion, but stopping at only eating one is a different matter entirely though.

Method:

Preheat your oven to 180C/160C Fan/350F/Gas mark 4. Lay out your whoopie pie tins and give them a light greasing before dusting them with flour.

Measure all of the wet ingredients into a mixing bowl then measure all of the dry ingredients into another bowl and give it a stir. Add the dry ingredients into the wet ingredients and mix well.

Pour equal amounts of the cake mix into the whoopie pie tins and bake in the oven for around 10-12 mins. (They're cooked if a skewer pushed into the middle of a couple of the cakes comes out entirely clean.)

Leave to cool before taking the whoopie pies out of the tin.

Place your buttercream ingredients in a large mixing bowl and whisk together. Once cool, sandwich the whoopie pies with the buttercream icing and serve.

Chocolate Orange Biscuits (Makes 8-10)

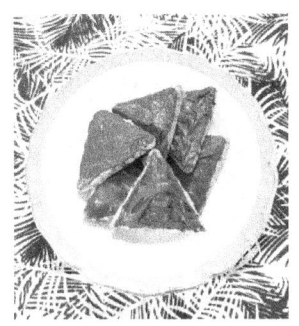

Ingredients:
70g butter (or dairy-free version)
30g coconut oil
80g gluten-free flour
20g cornflour
50g custard powder
70g caster sugar
The grated zest of 1 orange
1/2 tsp vanilla extract
1 tsp orange flavouring
1 tsp orange juice
1 tsp xanthan gum
1/2 tsp baking powder
200g dark chocolate (for the topping)

This chocolate orange biscuit recipe is really quick and easy to make and produces little crispy biscuits that are a doddle to top with melted chocolate. The inclusion of custard powder and a little bit of cornflour ensures that they have a good crunch, but still have a bit of crumble to them. I use a triangular cookie cutter which gives great results, but you can cut them out into any shape you like. The real struggle lies in waiting for the dark chocolate to cool and harden on the biscuits before you eat them. I'll bet you can't.

Method:

Preheat your oven to 200C/180C Fan/400F/Gas mark 6 and line two baking trays with greaseproof paper.

Melt the coconut oil and butter in a microwavable bowl then add all of the other ingredients and mix until a smooth dough is formed.

Roll out the dough onto a floured work surface and use the cookie cutter to cut your biscuits out and place them on the baking trays.

Bake the biscuits in the oven for 12 to 15 mins, or until they are golden brown. Remove from the oven and leave to cool.

Once the cookies are cold, melt the dark chocolate in a bowl in the microwave (stirring very frequently so that the chocolate doesn't burn).

Generously spread the chocolate over the cookies and leave to harden before serving. Or dive right in and get your chin and fingers covered in melted chocolate. It didn't happen to me, you understand, it was a friend one time…

Dark Chocolate And Ginger Oaties (Makes 12)

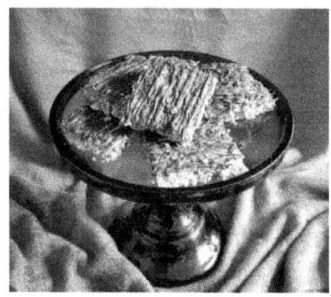

These dark chocolate and ginger oaties are crisp and sweet, but with the added deep flavour profile of the dark chocolate drizzle on top.

They're unbelievably easy and quick to make and keep in the biscuit tin for at least a week, if not more. It all depends on how much you can resist their tempting call.

One oatie is a low FODMAP portion.

Ingredients:
180g gluten-free oats
30g desiccated coconut
30g gluten-free flour
100ml melted coconut oil (or butter, if non-vegan)

1 tsp vanilla extract
30g sunflower seeds
30g pumpkin seeds
1 tsp xanthan gum
1 tbsp chia seeds soaked in 3 tbsp cold water for 1/2 an hour
1/2 cup dark brown sugar
1/2 tsp salt
2 tsps ground ginger
100g dark chocolate

Method:

Soak the chia seeds and then preheat your oven to 170C/150C Fan/350F/ Gas mark 4 and line a baking tin with greaseproof paper.

Melt the coconut oil and then put all of the ingredients into a large bowl and mix to combine. If you think the mixture is too dry just add some more coconut oil. (Sometimes oats can require more liquid.)

Tip the mixture into the baking tin and press it down before baking it in the oven for 25-30 minutes until golden brown.

Cut it into squares while it's still warm. Once your oaties have cooled down a bit, melt the dark chocolate and drizzle it over the oaties and leave to set. Wait until the biscuits are totally cold before removing from the baking tray.

Blondies (Makes 8-10)

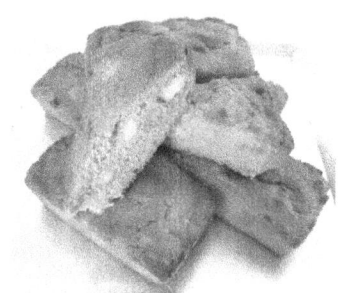

Ingredients:

350g sweet potato (peeled weight) cut into cubes
150g self-raising gluten-free flour
120g brown sugar
2 eggs
1 tsp vanilla
100g butter (or non-dairy)
1 tsp baking powder
100g dairy-free white chocolate chips
100g macadamia nuts
50ml rice milk

Blondies are very similar to brownies, but instead of using cocoa or dark or milk chocolate they are based around vanilla flavours, white chocolate and brown sugar. This combination of ingredients ensures that they remain lighter than their chocolate-laden brownie counterpart.

I use sweet potato in my blondie recipe because I think that incorporating the naturally sweet vegetable is a brilliant way to ensure that the bake remains soft and retains its moisture content.

Sweet potatoes are also an excellent source of fibre and B-vitamins, so it's a great way to include some nutrition within what is essentially a one-off treat!

If you prefer, you can substitute the macadamia nuts for the same weight in hazelnuts, brazil nuts, peanuts, pecans, pine nuts, pumpkin seeds or walnuts and they will remain low FODMAP.

One blondie is a low FODMAP serving.

Method:

Cook the sweet potato by peeling it and cutting it into small cubes and cooking it on a plate in the microwave until soft. Leave to cool.

Preheat your oven to 190C/170C Fan/375F/Gas mark 5.

Lay out your brownie cases on a baking tray. (You can use muffin cases instead, if you like.)

Put the butter and sugar in a mixing bowl and whisk until fluffy. Add the eggs, rice milk and vanilla and whisk again until combined.

Add the sweet potato, flour, baking powder and whisk until combined.

Fold the chocolate chips and macadamia nuts into the blondie mixture and divide between 8-10 brownie cases.

Bake for 25-30 mins or until a skewer pushed into the middle of them comes out clean. Leave to cool slightly and then serve.

Viennese Whirls (Makes 12)

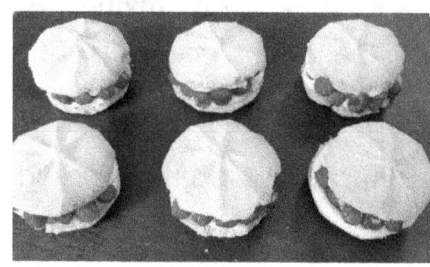

Viennese whirls are similar to empire biscuits, but they're much lighter and more delicate. Unlike empire biscuits, which are sandwiched solely with jam, Viennese whirls are sandwiched together with lightly whipped buttercream icing and strawberry jam which makes them a very sweet, but delightfully indulgent, treat. One Viennese whirl is a low FODMAP portion. Sometimes instead of jam I use fresh strawberries inside my Viennese whirls, but you can just use a low FODMAP strawberry jam instead.

Ingredients for the Viennese biscuits:

200g butter (or non-dairy)
50g icing sugar
1 tsp vanilla extract
180g plain flour

20g cornflour
1 tsp baking powder
1 tsp xanthan gum

Ingredients for the buttercream icing:

100g butter (or non-dairy)
180g icing sugar
3 tbsps of strawberry jam

Method:

Preheat your oven to 180C/160 Fan/350F/Gas Mark 5 and place greaseproof paper on a couple of baking trays.

Cream the butter, vanilla and icing sugar until fluffy and then add the flour, cornflour, baking powder and xanthan gum and mix well.

Put the mixture in a piping bag with a star-shaped nozzle and use the bag to pipe 5 cm circles onto the greaseproof paper, leaving a 3-4 cm gap between each.

Bake the biscuits for 10-14 mins until they are golden brown and then leave them to cool down. (They're extremely delicate, so just leave them on the baking tray to go completely cold before you take them off the trays.)

Make the buttercream by blending all of the ingredients together until smooth. Put it in a piping bag.

Once the biscuits are cold pipe buttercream around the rim of the bottom of each of the biscuits before putting a dollop of strawberry jam in the centre or adding fresh strawberries.

Sandwich the biscuits together and serve.

Red Velvet Muffins (Makes 12)

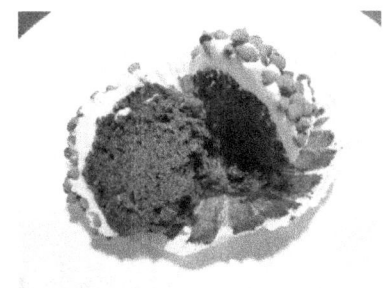

These red velvet muffins were created one day when I discovered that I had a tub of lactose-free cream cheese in the fridge which needed to be used up and I figured that it'd be a great topping for a red velvet cake. As much as I enjoy baking full size cakes, sometimes it's nice to make individual muffins because I find that they can stay soft and moist for longer. This is also helped by the addition of grated carrots which add a natural sweetness and help to keep the cake soft. It's quite simply the perfect muffin, in my humble opinion.

Ingredients for the muffins:

180g sugar

175ml vegetable oil
3 eggs
190g carrots (grated)
200g gluten-free flour
50g cocoa powder
1 tsp xanthan gum
1 tsp baking powder
1/2 tsp bicarbonate of soda
1 tsp vanilla extract
100ml rice milk
1 tsp red food colouring (optional)

Ingredients for the cream cheese frosting:

150g lactose-free cream cheese (or dairy-free)
100g icing sugar
1 tsp vanilla extract
Dark chocolate chips (to decorate)

Method:

Preheat your oven to 200C/180C Fan/400F/Gas Mark 6 and put 12 muffins cases in a muffin tray.

Mix all of the wet ingredients together in a large mixing bowl and then add all of the dry ingredients and mix well.

Divide equally between the 12 muffin cases and bake in the oven for 20-25 mins or until a skewer pushed into the middle of one comes out clean.

While the red velvet muffins are baking make the cream cheese frosting by mixing all of the frosting ingredients together in a bowl.

Once the muffins are done leave them to cool completely before topping them with the frosting and chocolate chips. Serve.

Strawberry Turnovers (Serves 8)

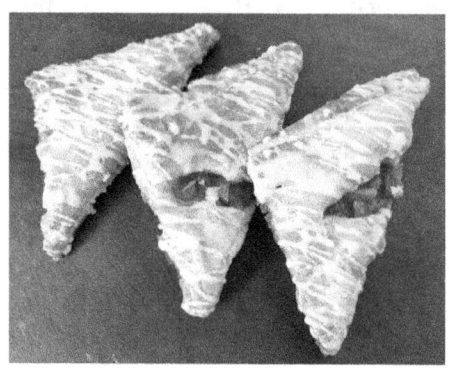

Strawberry turnovers are a refreshing and low FODMAP alternative to apple turnovers. They're really quick to make, but they're very rewarding in taste. I like to drizzle mine with a light layer of icing, but you can leave them plain, if you like, or even top them with melted chocolate. However you decide to adorn them you can be guaranteed it'll be a very tasty pastry!

Ingredients:
300g fresh strawberries (chopped)
500g gluten-free puff pastry
2 tbsps caster sugar
1 egg (beaten)
10 tbsps of icing sugar mixed with 4 tbsps of cold water

Method:

Preheat your oven to 200C/180C Fan/400F/Gas mark 6 and line a large baking tray with greaseproof paper.

Mix the chopped strawberries with the caster sugar in a bowl.

Roll out the puff pastry and cut it into 8 squares.

Place the strawberry mixture in the centre of each square of puff pastry and then brush beaten egg around the outside of each square before folding one edge of a puff pastry square over to the other forming a triangle. Place it on the greaseproofed baking tray.

Do the same with all of the turnovers and then bake them in the oven until the pastry is puffed and golden brown.

Coffee And Walnut Cake (Serves 8-10)

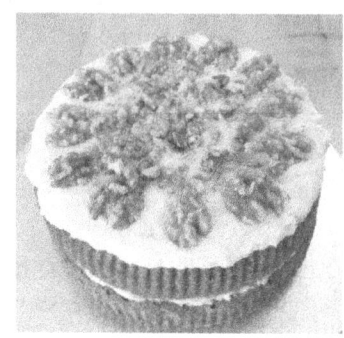

Ingredients for the coffee cake:

200g butter (or non-dairy)
200g sugar
4 eggs
1 tsp vanilla extract
2 tbsps instant coffee dissolved in 50ml of hot water
150g self-raising gluten-free flour
1 tsp baking powder
1 tsp xanthan gum

Ingredients for the buttercream icing:

200g butter (or non-dairy)
200g icing sugar
100g walnut halves

One of my favourite cakes is a coffee and walnut cake. I just love the flavour combination of deep, almost bitter, coffee and crunchy walnuts, especially when merged with sweet, whipped buttercream icing. This recipe makes a light and fluffy sponge cake that's got just the right level of coffee in it.

Method:

Preheat your oven to 180C/160 Fan/350F/Gas Mark 5 and line two 9 inch cake tins with greaseproof paper.

Dissolve the instant coffee in the hot water and leave it to cool.

Meanwhile, put the butter and sugar in a mixing bowl and whisk until fluffy.

Add the eggs, vanilla and coffee and whisk again until combined.

Add the flour, baking powder and xanthan gum and whisk until combined.

Divide the cake mixture between the two cake tins and bake in the oven for 30-35 mins or until a skewer pushed into the middle of the cakes comes out clean.

Leave the cakes to cool and make the buttercream icing in the meantime by mixing all of the icing ingredients together until combined.

Once the cake is cool, remove them from the cake tins and spread half of the buttercream on top of one cake and place the other cake on top.

Spread the rest of the buttercream on top of the cake and then decorate with the walnuts before serving.

www.ingramcontent.com/pod-product-compliance
Lightning Source LLC
Chambersburg PA
CBHW071440070526
44578CB00001B/166